FROM CURSED TO CURED

How to Treat & Cure PMDD Naturally

RACHEL LYNN FOX

Copyright © 2025 by Rachel Lynn Fox

All rights are reserved, and no part of this publication may be reproduced, distributed, or transmitted in any manner, whether through photocopying, recording, or any other electronic or mechanical methods, without the explicit prior written permission of the publisher. This restriction applies to any form or means of reproduction or distribution.

Exceptions to this rule include brief quotations that may be incorporated into critical reviews, as well as certain other noncommercial uses that are allowed by copyright law. Any such usage must adhere to the specified conditions and permissions outlined by the copyright holder.

Book Design by Hmdpublishing

PRAISE FOR RACHEL

"Absolutely life-changing, working with Rachel was incredible. I was slightly skeptical in the beginning about what was achievable because I was at such a low point, but in the end, my symptoms, on a scale of 0-10, went from 8, 9, and 10 to 0. I have never felt so aligned, capable, and motivated. I gained an immense amount of self-understanding that I know will have a lifelong positive effect. I feel unrecognizable compared to four months ago and am so very, very grateful! Thank you endlessly, Rachel!" - AJ T

"My journey with Rachel has truly changed my life. I've been suffering from PMDD since I was 13 (about five years now) and had never been able to find a fix. I tried doctors, medications, therapy, and vitamins, but nothing ever gave me enough relief until I started working with Rachel. She is so incredibly sweet, compassionate, understanding, flexible, and knowledgeable. The program is completely tailored to what you want to improve on, and Rachel is constantly there for questions and to be a resource as well as a cheerleader. She is such a beautiful soul." - Ashley Blum

"Rachel has changed my world. I was at the lowest point and thought no one could help me after countless doctor appointments and countless awful, horrible days and thoughts & being told, 'Go on birth control.' Rachel's RTT sessions are immensely strong and powerful. The whole entire process is a miracle and magical. There are not enough words of amazingness I could say about Rachel and this program. You must be committed and fully want that change – and if you do – you will feel the most amazing shift & become YOU again and FREE!" - Anita Cimera

"I honestly don't even know where to begin when it comes to expressing my gratitude for Rachel! I've been working with Rachel for the past four months in her Living in Luteal program and to say it's changed my life is an understatement! I had no idea what PMDD was up until a few months prior to finding Rachel. I have been dealing with pretty severe PMDD symptoms for most of my life, but I didn't know what it was from. Thankfully, I came across a week-long PMDD summit that was taking place on Facebook. I watched every single interview with many different PMDD experts, but as soon as I saw Rachel's interview, I knew she was the person I needed to reach out to! Honestly, I was a little bit hesitant and nervous because I was really scared it wouldn't work for me because so many things I have tried in the past have failed. I decided to listen to my gut instead and start the program with Rachel! Thank goodness I did because, at the beginning of the program, I was not in a good place at all. I was depressed, angry, hopeless, filled with fear, fatigued, binge eating, and had zero confidence, just to name a few. Today, I have done a complete 180! I have so much energy, am so positive, and my confidence has been restored! I owe this all to Rachel! I no longer have any of my PMDD symptoms, plus she has helped me in so many other areas of my life! I am forever grateful and I'm looking forward to continuing to work with her in the future! She is the kindest, most caring person I've ever met! A true healer! Thank you, Rachel" - April Nygaard

"I can't say enough good things about Rachel and her program. She worked with my daughter, and Rachel was the first person she was able to open up to and really helped her work through her feelings. Rachel has been wonderful for my daughter!" - Amybeth Travis

"I had never done hypnotherapy or RTT before reaching out to Rachel. It's hard to consolidate what a transformative time the last four months have been in a short blurb, but Rachel is a wonderful person, hypnotherapist, and coach. Despite my hesitancy to try a new framework of healing, I knew I couldn't continue to live in the type of cyclical pain I was suffering from with PMDD. I've had different points in time where PMDD was more manageable on SSRIs, but I had a recent health flare-up that made me have to take a break from all medication. My PMDD was the worst it had ever been for the months leading up to finding Rachel. I wanted to experience life to the fullest that my body could offer off of medicine, and something in the cosmos allowed me to find Rachel! I noticed a huge shift after the first RTT session; these sessions allowed me to unpack decades of trauma that, honestly, I just couldn't get at in traditional talk therapy. The only sad thing about this whole process was that I didn't find it sooner, but I'm so grateful for the healing work Rachel facilitated. PMDD is a hard, hard thing to live with, and if you've tried everything else and nothing has worked, try working with Rachel! What I told myself going in was, at the very least, I'll have four months of working on myself, dedicating time to healing, and hopefully moving through some trauma. What I got was a total absence of PMDD and even a healthier, more joyous mindset in the weeks outside of PMDD, as it really affects the whole month in terms of stress and cyclical repeating trauma for the body and mind. Rachel made me feel super comfortable and held, and she has a clear calling to this, frankly, lifesaving work. My PMDD is just no longer there; it has just literally gone away. I'll be forever grateful. If you're not sure whether or not to try this and you have PMDD, just do it." - Sam Tabet

"Rachel's 'Living in Luteal' program was life-changing. Having struggled with PMDD for so many years, I am amazed at how quickly I was able to let it all go. There was definitely an extra level of comfort I had with Rachel, given she has also healed from PMDD, which is typically not the case with other professionals. She is so knowledgeable and has such a calm and supportive energy. I cannot recommend her enough!" - Amy Feldhacker

"I spent a decade trying to find a diagnosis. I didn't want to keep living with chronic pain and fatigue. It was robbing me of so much. Finally, finding out I had PMDD and gaining the knowledge that there was a treatment that could set me free brought tears to my eyes. Hope finally returned. Four months later, after completing Rachel's program, I just had my first luteal phase symptom-free in over a decade... I can't begin to explain how amazing this is. My relationships with my kids are better, I'm active, I have an interest in my hobbies again, and I have energy for life! There is hope. There is healing for PMDD." - Holly Remaly

"I can't really explain the depths of the changes within me over the last three months while working with Rachel, but I will do my best. After over a decade of being a holistic therapist myself and trying many different modalities of healing and therapies, working with Rachel has been the most profound and healing experience I have gotten the chance to go through, and I am forever grateful to Rachel for her empathy, wisdom, and dedication to this transformational process. I found Rachel when I was at my absolute worst, with nothing left, debilitating mood swings, and panic attacks, all stemming from childhood trauma, expressing itself in the form of PMDD. As soon as we met, my hopes began to rise, and this process became my 24/7 job. To keep it short, each hypnotherapy session was a deep dive into moments and memories that shaped my unconscious reactions to life today. With her calm voice and knowledge in the field, we were able to go back to the moments and heal from that point forward. Each hypnotherapy session was like a soul boost of compassion, strength, and understanding from deep within. The weekly therapy meetings with Rachel were perfectly placed, and she was readily available anytime I needed some extra support. On a scale from one to ten (ten being the worst), I began this process with a 10. Three months later, I am at a 0. For the first time in my life, I truly feel the best I have ever felt inside of myself. Authentically myself. I feel strong, brave, safe, calm, clear, and ready to move forward in a way that I only dreamed of before. I am able to speak and live my truth without doubt. The deep-seated pain I had felt and pushed down my entire life has been replaced with hope and clarity. I am forever grateful to Rachel for coming into my life, and I will always carry everything I learned during this process with me. I have become the best version of myself for me...my family, partner, friends, and clients. Thank you from the bottom of my heart and soul. If you have found Rachel, there is a reason for it. Follow your intuition! 10 out of 10" - Emily Williams

"After completing Living in Luteal: Self-Guided Experience. I knew I wanted more! I needed more! Being a natural self-reflector, learner, and thinker, I craved it. When the opportunity arose for me to continue by taking a four-month deeper dive into my self-healing quest, I just had to. With PMDD and a lifelong trauma history, including a rare genetic syndrome, I was beyond excited to continue working in the program. I was more committed and determined than ever, doing the hard work daily. There were so many tears. Tears of grief... Tears of relief... and, more importantly, Tears of pride. Even during the most challenging moments, Rachel was by my side! She always met me wherever I was in those moments. At the same time, when I was ready, she was not afraid to challenge me.

As I officially completed. Living in the Luteal 4-Month Program, I know that my journey is not over; it is just the beginning. It is beyond mind-blowing to think about where I was just seven months ago when the universe brought Rachel and RTT into my life. It is evident to those closest to and around me that I am coming out of hiding, out from behind the shadows... becoming the person I am meant to be. I'm eternally grateful for our RTT. I am even more excited to be able to continue sharing my journey and life experiences, as well as to give back to those who have supported me the most.

I cannot thank Rachel enough for all her guidance and support. Her passion and belief in those she works with clearly show as we share our personal experiences along the way, which is part of the process. Through tears and laughter... Because she just gets it! Having that type of person holding my hand through this journey over the past seven months has been crucial. Rachel is not only an amazing mentor but a very dear friend. I'm excited to see our paths continue to cross in the future. As one lasting thought, as I continue to heal every moment of every day, I see the love behind the compliments that others give me, and I am finally seeing what they have always seen in me while also finding who I was always meant to be." - Tara Lynne Ethier-Southard.

DEDICATED TO

To my daughters Naomi & Ella:
You are both my why, my reason for everything.

To my husband, John:
Who could see the real me, and who waited for me to come back home.

To my parents:
Thank you for being an example of faith and
showing me the path to know God.

FORWARD

I am pleased to introduce this book by Rachel Lynn Fox, which explores healing from Premenstrual Dysphoric Disorder (PMDD) using Rapid Transformational Therapy (RTT). Rachel's approach focuses on addressing the root causes of PMDD, offering a pathway to relief and recovery.

PMDD, or Premenstrual Dysphoric Disorder, is a condition that affects many individuals, often disrupting their lives in significant ways. In this book, Rachel draws upon her personal experience and professional expertise to offer a clear and compassionate guide to healing. By using RTT, she addresses the underlying issues that contribute to PMDD, providing a path toward recovery.

Rachel's approach is practical, rooted in her understanding of the mind, and dedicated to helping others find relief and reclaim their lives. This book is a valuable resource for anyone seeking to overcome PMDD.

Marisa Peer
Founder of RTT

CONTENTS

1. A Journey Through Shadows 10
2. Let's Get Educated. Period. 20
3. Understanding PMDD. 39
4. Becoming Unstuck in an Endless Cycle of Chaos 59
5. The Road Less Traveled.. 71
6. Your Sensitivity is a Gift 98
7. Decoding Sensitivity, Understanding Triggers 108
8. The Deep Dive 119
9. Your Higher Identity & Self is Calling 141

Appendix. 172

About the Author 188

Chapter ONE

A JOURNEY THROUGH SHADOWS

I was born and raised in a Christian home where love and faith were the foundations of our lives. My parents are still married and live in the same home my older sister, younger brother and I grew up in, providing us a stable and nurturing environment. We prayed together and went to church every Sunday, and our home was filled with the warmth of family dinners and gatherings grounded in Biblical truths.

My father, a hard-working, successful entrepreneur, started a home security business with my uncle in 1972. There were always talks of making sure our home was secure, protected, and safe from essentially bad people. We grew up with the belief that the world was a place of wonder and opportunity, yet we were also taught to be mindful that not everyone had good intentions or could be fully trusted. Growing up in the 80s, I remember eating my bowl of cereal in the morning, staring at the milk carton with the kidnap inscription along the side of the container. I always read it. A childhood fear quickly became the fear of being kidnapped. And it was ingrained in me, "Do not talk to strangers."

It turns out that 1983 was a particularly impactful year for me. I was just six years old when my father led a large church split, exposing the head pastor with morally hidden sins. The day we were kicked out of our church and told never to return, I remember hearing a lot of men yelling and screaming. My parents, sister, and I were escorted out the front doors; the pastor's wife physically pushed my mom out the front door while she was pregnant with my brother. I blurted out, "Don't touch my mom!" We walked across the parking lot and climbed into our Oldsmobile Cutlass to drive the next 30 minutes in almost silence; my dad told my sister and me that he would explain all of this to us when we were older. My mom cried all the way home. I remember wondering on that drive home, why were we kicked out? Does this mean God is mad at me and my family? If He is, does He still love us, does He still love me?

During that same summer of 1983, my family and my uncle's family all drove to the Jersey Shore for the day. I was the youngest of my four cousins and sister when we took a long walk along the beach. My cousins and sister stopped to watch a game that some kids were playing in the water. At the same time, I also stopped and turned and saw a girl building a sandcastle. What seemed like just a moment, I turned to look over at my family, and I did not see them. I began to turn in every direction, looking for them, but I could not see them. Everything began to look the same. I began to panic. Suddenly, I found myself lost on a hot and crowded beach for hours. Terrified and crying, I ran as far as I could in one direction, looking for them. I must have run the wrong way. So, I ran in the opposite direction as far as I could. I still did not see them. I ran up and down the beach until my legs couldn't take me any further. Thoughts that I might never see my family again began to sink in. Was I going to be kidnapped? Would my family find me? Was I forgotten? Did they leave me on purpose? Am I going to get in trouble? I fell on my knees, collapsed in the sand and just started crying when an older woman came up to me and asked if I was lost. I looked up at her, wiping the tears from my eyes, nodding my head, and told her I was not supposed to talk to strangers. She invited me to sit on her blanket while her husband went to report me missing to the lifeguards. I sat at the very edge of the blanket, holding my knees to my chest, when suddenly, I heard my aunt's voice, she was screaming my name, I ran to her and hugged her, sobbing; I was joyfully reunited with my parents who affectionately covered me in hugs and kisses. Those hours and that event ended up leaving a deep impression on me and in me.

At the end of that summer, my baby brother was born. While this was a celebratory time in our home, it marked a significant transition for me. I had to give up my bedroom as it became my brother's nursery, which meant I had to share a room and a full-size bed with my older sister, who was nine years old at the time. I lost my own space and all the things that having my own room represented to me, while I also felt like I was invading my sister's room. We fought a lot. I bothered her a lot, understandably. Our arguments often sounded like, "Find your own place," "Get out," and "Leave me alone; this was my room first." We shared her room for the next six years.

Maybe it was because all these things happened so close to each other, but I remember feeling and noticing for the first time that I was extremely sensitive. I felt like there was a lot of confusion, frustration, a ton of fear, and a lot of tears. My tears were often misunderstood. I often heard things like "You are such a cry-baby," "Why are you always crying?" "You turn on tears like a spicket." "What's wrong with you?" "Suck it up," and "You need to grow tougher skin." I remember feeling like my emotions were too big for me. I was often easily hurt; I didn't know how to hide the huge heart that was on my sleeve.

From kindergarten to eighth grade, I attended a Christian school. I remember experiencing my first taste of rejection when my kindergarten crush chose another girl to sit next to during reading time. I thought to myself, "I wish I had blonde hair; that would make me prettier." In elementary school, I was teased because of my freckles. Inspired by the book *Freckle Juice*, I once mixed all our refrigerator condiments and rubbed them on my skin, hoping to wake up without those little spots. The next morning, I was disappointed to find my freckles still there. That feeling of wanting what I could not have, of longing for the prettier frame, hair, skin and looks, stayed with me.

As I moved into middle school, I became increasingly self-conscious about my appearance and developed an extremely poor body image. To cope, I secretly bought laxatives from the pharmacy up the street from my house. If I could just lose some extra pounds, everything would be better. Then came the day that many of us young women remember vividly—the day we got our period. It happened during gym class, and I ran to the bathroom, embarrassed and terrified, and decided that hiding in the bathroom for the rest of the day was a better option than returning to class, fearing that I would be teased or laughed at.

Although I was active in sports, played the flute and piano, and had the lead vocal solos in our holiday and spring performances, I was deeply insecure. I thought this insecurity was just a part of growing up, but it weighed heavily on me, shaping my self-perception and sense of worth.

Attending public high school was my chance to spread my wings. I wanted to make a good impression and wanted to be liked, like any other new student. I joined the theater, all the choirs, soccer team, and the high school marching band. I loved being a part of it all. Beyond the extracurricular activities, I found & still have to this day, a lifelong, loyal, ride-or-die girl group who stood by me through my first real relationship with my boyfriend and my first heartbreak that followed. The knife-like pain of betrayal and rejection was epitomized by Alanis Morissette's "You Oughta Know," which we belted out with the windows down in my Ford Station Wagon, affectionately known as the El Segundo. The anger that began surfacing seemed very justified and even validating. Yet, even from my closest clique, I tried to hide my depression, my struggles with laxatives, my tumultuous relationship with food, the cycles of binging and purging, and my deeply ingrained horrible body image issues.

During my junior and senior years, my childhood dream began to appear in my heart: I wanted to sing. I aspired to be a professional singer, and after all the years and countless hours of voice lessons my parents had paid for, I was determined to put these gifts and talents to use. So, when it was time to apply to colleges, it seemed natural to declare to my parents and family that I was going to major in vocal performance.

Singing brought me back to life. Music kept me alive. I found expression and release, and it was my own. But when I shared my plans with my parents, my hopes and dreams felt crushed. My father, who was graciously paying for my education, suggested that I minor in vocal music to ensure I had a good career to fall back on. It *felt* like my heart cracked in two. Although I understood his desire for me to have a "safe" plan, it *felt* like he did not believe in me, that he did not think I was good enough. It *felt* like he thought I just was not that talented.

So, accepting this as my harsh reality, I swallowed that jagged little pill. I was angered, I was hurting, and I longed to get to college where I could finally be free. While all my older cousins and sister attended a Christian university, I was determined to pave my own path. During the next few years in college in Virginia, I decided to experience life to the fullest, and I did just that. I tried a lot of new things: I got my first tattoo, I self-medicated a lot, I went to my first concerts and festivals, fell in love with vintage clothing, I met many great people and professors, and also transferred schools to New York, all in pursuit of happiness and really what I wanted. I immersed myself in a season of self-exploration through every means possible. Yet, amidst all these experiences, I knew I was grappling with a very dark undercurrent of pain. No matter what I did or how hard I tried, how hard I prayed, I could not outrun the thoughts in my head and what felt like feelings of darkness within me.

The desperation for relief drove me to seek God, I became exhausted in my own soul-searching. I started going to a church that was within walking distance of my apartment. My roots, faith, and the prayers of my grandmother and parents led me to a profound spiritual encounter one evening at a young adult service. I knew that something had dramatically shifted in me; there was happiness, peace, and a lightness in my mind. I felt better, and the depression didn't seem so dark. I called my parents that night to tell them about my experience. It was an answer to prayer, it felt miraculous. It was also at this time I was presented with a massive opportunity that would have changed my life forever, I was offered a deal to sign with a major record label. I could not believe what was happening. The label's only conditions were that I would have to cut my hair, wear tight clothing, and put out a very sexy image since that is what the industry needed. I was shocked and horrified that these were the demands. I felt like if I agreed to this, I would be literally selling my soul. So, I said no. I could not believe that after all the years of wanting this, it was coming up now.

During that spring break, a group from this church invited me to attend a three-day youth revival conference in Florida. I went, and it was life-changing for me. It was then that I felt a call to ministry. I wrapped up my third year of college and found myself that summer on a three-week mission's trip to Venezuela; I honestly considered not returning home. I wanted purpose. I really wanted to figure out my next steps and what God had for me. During this season, while attending another conference, I met a Christian guy who wanted to serve God the same way I did. Our six-month long-distance relationship had us eagerly applying to a very radical school of ministry in the South (connected to the same youth conference that I had just attended.) We were both accepted. Quickly, we found out that there were some very strict rules regarding hanging out with the opposite sex. It was not accepted. It was forbidden. We understood the rules to mean that if you were engaged, you would be allowed to go on dates and have time to just get to know one another. So, we decided to start our first spring semester engaged. (Even though we came to find out, we were not permitted to be alone, even as an engaged couple.) During this time, we were strongly encouraged in our pre-marital classes and by leadership to get married to avoid sexual sin, so after one semester, we got married; I just turned 22. We were happy, we were in God's will and in love, we were serving the Lord while earnestly desiring God's plan to unfold in our lives. Despite all the new exciting beginnings and being part of the music and worship teams, prayer groups, and evangelical teams at the school, I often felt like a poster child for condemnation. I could not escape the suffering of my thoughts and feelings like I was never enough or doing enough. I carried shame, and soon, that familiar tidal wave of plummeting self-esteem overtook me, pulling me under. That dark depression and the critical body image issues returned. The feelings of rejection and unworthiness felt more intense as well. Despite my prayers, fasting, Bible classes, studies, singing on worship teams, my relationship with God, ministry work, and being a wife, there was a void inside of me. I started questioning if God loved me, if something was wrong with me, if there was a crucial chemical missing in my brain, if I was cursed.

We graduated, and we both became ordained ministers and for most of our 19 years of marriage, we served in the ministry. We traveled abroad, taking short-term mission trips to several countries in Europe and Israel, and worked alongside local churches in Alabama, Florida, New York, and Pennsylvania while having two beautiful daughters along the way. Like all marriages, we had our highs and lows; we had our disagreements, arguments, and our times of joy and laughter. Some words landed deeper than others, producing scars on top of pre-existing wounds. I soon noticed the cavern of pain was getting deeper, rejection and darkness filled my chest too often. I found myself unhappy, stuck, resentful, bitter, alone and angered, feeling more than half of every month swallowed up in feelings of deep sadness, hopelessness, and questioning my life and purpose. There were many times I would get down on my hands and knees on the floor in my kitchen, begging, pleading in agony to God to please take the pain away from me. I was so embarrassed and so ashamed that I was not strong enough to fight it like a good, strong woman of God.

I knew deep in my heart that I really could not go on for much longer like this, and after pursuing our emerging professional careers in our final attempt to save our marriage while taking a break from ministry in California, we mutually agreed it was time to separate. The decision was not easy; my family was not supportive of it, it came with much fear, isolation, and immense emotional pain, but I was so weary and so tired; it just wasn't healthy for me, it wasn't healthy for him, but most importantly it wasn't healthy for our precious daughters who deserved so much more.

We decided to move back to the east coast. Suddenly, I was a single mom in Manhattan, raising two teenage daughters. I was overwhelmed but determined. Although I continued to battle the emotional rollercoaster, by the grace of God, over the next several years, I advanced my way up the ladder in luxury retail management, but a very toxic relationship overshadowed my achievements. After 18 months of dating a complete narcissist, tormented by emotional and physical abuse by a guy that I met through an acquaintance, the relationship ended; I was filled with shame, humiliation, and embarrassment. Looking back, I see how I attracted him. Narcissists prey on low self-esteem by exploiting insecurities, gaslighting them, manipulating the vulnerable person's need for validation, and using this dependency to gain control and power over them. And although it was the healthiest thing I could do to end the relationship, just like that, all my beliefs resurrected again, confirming that I was not lovable, I was not enough, I was not meant to know love, I just was not going to know happiness…it just was not available for me.

Being encouraged by my daughters, friends, and family, I redirected my energy inward; I had to dig deep, and I began to realign with my values and my faith, creating better boundaries and connecting deeper to the love that was in our apartment of three. A year later, I thought I was ready for a new relationship, he was a kind and generous man, he had his baggage and apparently, I had a U-Haul. Relationships bring out your very best and your worst. With the newness of love, joy, and laughter, I also began to quickly notice my old destructive reoccurring life themes resurfacing with more frequency: the trust issues, jealousy, being easily irritated and bothered, having a severe sensitivity to rejection, and when I could no longer contain the brewing intense emotions an uncontrollable explosion of anger would erupt.

I could not believe this was happening to me again, and it felt even worse. After all this time and all the prayers, getting back into the church, and the attempts of trying to become better, UGH, nothing, I guess, stuck. All I saw in the mirror was this horrible, ugly monster. Days following these angry outbursts, I was humiliated, I was defeated, and I would cry and beg for forgiveness from my daughters, my boyfriend, and even friends or family that I might have offended. This became my normal, my sick, sick normal.

It was right about then that COVID-19 hit I watched the world change and my life. I lost my job, and my daughter's private school closed completely, including remote learning. My mental, physical, and spiritual health deteriorated rapidly.

For the next year, I felt like I was losing the battle. I masked and hid my struggles outside of my home the best I could, confiding in my general doctor, endocrinologist, ob-gyn, and therapists. I told them that I was experiencing depression and anxiety. But could I really tell them how bad it was without sounding completely psycho?! If I told them how bad it was at times, could they be trusted, would it be reported, would I lose my kids?

I needed help I needed relief. I had hormonal tests run and blood work drawn; everything was coming back normal. I felt like I was dying inside—this cannot be normal!! Over that next year, I was prescribed anti-depressants and anti-anxiety medications, I eliminated gluten and alcohol, I was taking supplements, working out, and even tried ketamine therapy. Yet, I was still suffering in ways I was too ashamed to speak about. The side effects from the medications had me feeling even more chaotic. My depression and rage reached an all-time high I began to wonder if I was bipolar. After every episode, I would promise my boyfriend and my daughters that I was going to get this under control and that these kinds of outbursts were never going to happen again. I kept promising them.

Then, one night, everything skyrocketed. I lost it. My boyfriend left me and jumped on the first flight to Florida he could find. Devastated, I had to look into the eyes of my daughters, full of shame, horror, and sorrow. I told myself that night they would be better off without me. They deserved a better mom. I was unrecognizable. All night long, I just kept crying; the pain was inconsolable. I contemplated taking my life. That next morning, blanketed in shame, I grabbed my laptop. I needed answers, and it was then, like I heard God speaking through me, that I googled "rage before period," and for the first time, I read three words that would change my life forever: Premenstrual Dysphoric Disorder, known as PMDD.

I could not believe what I began to read. I could not believe that I was just learning about this at the age of 44; I had never heard of this before. Everything I read was describing exactly what I was experiencing. Turning to YouTube, in tears of relief, I spent hours watching video after video; there were women all over the world who were suffering just like me. I was not alone. I was not crazy. I was not bipolar. I was not a monster. There was a name. I texted some of the videos to my boyfriend in hopes that he would respond since we had not communicated since the big blowout. About an hour later, he FaceTimed me back, and with tears streaming down both of our faces, he said "Babe, this is you. This is exactly it. This describes you to a T. What can you do? What is helping this? What are the next steps?" From there, I joined every PMDD Facebook support group I could find, feeling immediate validation. Again, for hours, I read post after post, but suddenly, my validation and my relief turned to complete dread. Every suggestion and every piece of advice that was being shared in all of these groups, I had tried. I could feel the dark cloud sweeping me back under. I began to read there was not a cure, and the only real answer was surgery. Removing parts of my body?! The cure was a complete hysterectomy, removing my uterus, cervix, and both ovaries. WHAT?!?! In addition, I would have to prove a long history of PMDD to my doctors before they would consider me for approval. I closed my laptop, and I just cried. Personally, for me, surgery was not something I was going to consider. I was defeated, I was terrified, and hope was gone. For days, I searched and scrolled for answers online, and I was led back to the support groups. I kept reading post after post, drilling down into comments…something in me told me to keep looking, just keep searching, do not give up….

My relentless determination led me to learn that some WERE finding relief, some even said they were HEALED, and some said that they were FREED and CURED from PMDD through a proven science-based approach. Finally, there was HOPE!

All along, I realized I was only trying to treat my symptoms. It did not occur to me that I was seeking to treat the root cause, nor did I understand that that was even possible. Isn't it interesting to think that we are not taught that? I began to read and learn that I could explore the root cause of my symptoms instead of just managing them. This is the moment everything changed; it was my game changer, my AHA! moment. This is when my deep healing journey of self-discovery and restoration began. I was determined and committed to doing the work, whatever it was, I was all in.

Now, my heart's desire is to share this journey with you. Here is the absolute truth, a truth that you will not hear out in our world. There is hope, there is healing, and there is freedom from the debilitating destruction of PMDD.

From this place of a renewed life, having a renewed family, and that boyfriend who left me is now my husband, and now having been restored back to my identity, purpose, and service, it is my prayer that this book will awaken in you your truth. May it stir something deep within you, resonating with the parts of you that have felt lost, unheard, and unseen. As you read this, may you find the courage to embark on your own journey of healing and reclaim your life from the shadows of PMDD.

You are not alone in this struggle. There is a path to freedom, and it begins with understanding, compassion, and a willingness to seek out the root causes of your pain. Let this book be a beacon of hope, guiding you toward self-awareness and self-understanding, leading toward wholeness and inner peace. My prayer is that through these pages, you will find the strength to confront your struggles, the wisdom to seek healing, and the grace to embrace your true self. There is hope for a brighter tomorrow, and it starts with believing in your own worth and the possibility of change.

Chapter Two

LET'S GET EDUCATED. PERIOD.

> *"Menstruation is not a curse it is a gift that allows us to connect with our bodies and the earth in a profound way."*
> **- Period Power**

Where do we begin? It must start with a conversation most of us have never had—a topic so taboo, so "dirty," so understudied, so under-researched, and so often swept under the carpet in our societies. Until now, it most likely is not discussed in our homes, in our schools, or, God forbid, in our churches. So, it is here that we must begin the discussion on understanding our menstrual cycles.

The menstrual cycle, a natural and integral part of every single woman's life, has long been shrouded in silence and stigma. This lack of open dialogue and comprehensive education has left most women unaware of the profound insights our bodies offer.

From a young age, many women are introduced to menstruation in a purely biological context, often without a deeper understanding of its cyclical nature and its connection to our overall health. Schools may touch on the basics of menstruation in sex education classes, but the intricate interplay between hormones, emotions, and physical well-being is rarely discussed.

I was 44 years old when I first learned, through my own online research, that there are four phases in our menstrual cycle. Did you know that? I remember asking my teenage daughters if they were taught this, and of course, they were not. I asked friends and family, and NO ONE KNEW! How has this been so overlooked in our education? This massive knowledge gap has profound implications, particularly when it comes to recognizing and addressing premenstrual disorders like PMDD.

PMDD, characterized by severe emotional and physical symptoms during the luteal phase of the menstrual cycle, is often misunderstood or misdiagnosed. Many women endure years of suffering, attributing their symptoms to personal flaws or unrelated health issues. This misattribution stems from a lack of awareness about how the menstrual cycle can influence one's mental and physical state.

By bringing awareness to the menstrual cycle and its phases, we can detect early signs and signals that the mind and body are communicating. This awareness is not merely about tracking periods but involves understanding the hormones and the cyclical changes in mood, energy levels, and physical sensations. Educating women, young girls, and AFAB (assigned female at birth) about these patterns can empower us to recognize when something is amiss.

Imagine a world where young girls are taught to understand and listen to their bodies, recognizing that the emotional changes they experience are not signs of weakness but signals that their bodies are expressing their needs. This education would foster empowerment, self-care and encourage proactive healthcare, helping to reduce the stigma and shame often linked to premenstrual symptoms.

Menstrual cycle education can foster a supportive community where women and AFAB share their experiences and insights, reducing the isolation many feel. It creates an environment where seeking help is normalized, and early intervention becomes the norm rather than the exception.

Incorporating menstrual cycle education into our broader health curriculum is not just a step towards gender equality but a profound shift toward holistic health and well-being for all menstruators. It acknowledges that understanding our bodies is a fundamental right, and this knowledge serves as a powerful tool in managing and understanding women's health issues. By advocating for comprehensive menstrual cycle education, we are not merely educating; we are empowering.

Expanding on this importance, it is essential to recognize how this knowledge can transform the lives of women and AFAB individuals. When equipped with an understanding of their menstrual cycles, they gain the ability to interpret the nuanced messages their bodies send throughout the month. This education is a beacon of hope, illuminating a path where early detection and proactive management of premenstrual disorders like PMDD become possible. We are equipping individuals with the tools to live in harmony with their cycles, free from the shadows of misunderstanding and neglect.

THE MENSTRUAL CYCLE: A SHARED GLOBAL EXPERIENCE

Believe it or not, at any given moment, around 300 million women worldwide are sharing a common experience—menstruation, or as it is more casually known, having a period. This universal rite of passage typically kicks off for young women or AFAB between the ages of 8 and 15 and wraps up around age 50 when menopause comes knocking. The average woman will ovulate about 300 to 400 times throughout her lifetime, resulting in quite a few menstrual cycles.

THE U.S. PERSPECTIVE

There are roughly 166 million women in the United States, and about 64 million of them are in the menstruating age range of 12-49. That's a lot of menstrual products and chocolate cravings!

10 MENSTRUAL CYCLE FACTS FOR THE U.S.

1. **Lifetime Supply**: The average American woman will have about 450 periods in her lifetime, which is roughly 6.25 years of menstruation!
2. **Tampon Count:** A woman might use between 11,000 and 16,000 tampons or pads over her lifetime, which is enough to build a small mountain of menstrual products.
3. **Hormonal Symphony**: Each month, your body conducts an intricate hormonal symphony, with estrogen, progesterone, FSH, and LH

all taking turns in the spotlight. It's like having a rock concert in your ovaries!

4. **Cycle Length**: While the average menstrual cycle is about 28 days, cycles ranging from 21 to 35 days are perfectly normal. Think of it as your personal biological rhythm.
5. **Menstrual Products** Market: The U.S. menstrual products market is worth over $3 billion annually. That's a lot of pads, tampons, and menstrual cups!
6. **First Period Age**: The average age for a girl to get her first period in the U.S. is around 12, though it can vary widely from 8 to 15.
7. **PMS Prevalence**: Approximately 75% of women experience some form of premenstrual syndrome (PMS), which can include mood swings, bloating, and cramps.
8. **Eco-Friendly Choices**: Menstrual cups and reusable pads are becoming increasingly popular in the U.S., with more women seeking eco-friendly alternatives to traditional disposable products.
9. **Period Poverty:** Around 1 in 5 girls in the U.S. have missed school due to a lack of access to menstrual products. This has sparked many initiatives to provide free menstrual supplies in schools.
10. **Menstrual Leave**: Although not common, a few progressive companies in the U.S. are starting to offer menstrual leave policies, recognizing the impact of menstrual symptoms on productivity and well-being.

These facts highlight the significant impact and ongoing conversations around menstrual health in the U.S., from market trends to social issues and individual experiences. Whether you are navigating the aisles of menstrual products or calculating the next time Aunt Flo will visit, it is all part of this global experience. So next time you reach for that heating pad or that extra bar of chocolate, remember you are in good company—millions of women worldwide are right there with you. This shared journey, filled with its own rhythms and nuances, is a testament to the beauty and power of the menstrual cycle, inspiring and empowering us in a profound and universal sisterhood.

GETTING TO KNOW THE PHASES OF THE MENSTRUAL CYCLE

Understanding the menstrual cycle phases is a journey into the profound interplay between our bodies, minds, and spirits. Each phase of the cycle—the menstruation, follicular, ovulation, and luteal phases—brings distinct hormonal shifts, emotional responses, and physical sensations. By breaking down each phase, we will explore when it occurs, its duration, the hormonal dynamics at play, and the scientific processes unfolding within the body. We will also delve into the emotional landscape that accompanies each phase, connecting these changes to the seasons and lunar cycles.

This understanding is not just about education; it is about reclaiming our power and deepening our connection to the natural rhythms that govern our lives. By learning this, we can better navigate our menstrual cycles, fostering a holistic sense of well-being that honors the intricate connections between mind, body, and spirit.

Understanding the menstrual cycle's connection to the seasons and lunar cycles offers insights into the natural rhythms that govern our lives. Each phase of the menstrual cycle mirrors the stages of the seasons and the phases of the moon, providing a deeper connection to the natural world and our intrinsic biological patterns.

Early menstruators often aligned their cycles with the moon, using its phases to understand and predict their menstrual patterns. This ancient wisdom recognized the moon's influence on the natural world, including tides, plant growth, and human biology. Women gathered in "moon lodges" or "red tents" to honor their cycles, create rituals, and support one another during menstruation, fostering a deep sense of community and spiritual connection. Let's begin…

MENSTRUATION - THEME INNER WINTER

Duration: Approximately 3-7 days
Days: Day 1 to Day 5-7 of the cycle

What hormonally is going on:

- ✧ Estrogen and Progesterone: Both hormones are at their lowest levels. The decrease in these hormones signals the body to start shedding the uterine lining, marking the start of menstruation.

✧ Follicle-Stimulating Hormone (FSH): Begins to rise to prepare for the next cycle. FSH stimulates the growth of ovarian follicles for the next round of ovulation.

What are some physical and emotional responses you might experience:

✧ Physical: Cramping, fatigue, breast tenderness, bloating, and headaches are common. These symptoms result from the body's effort to shed the uterine lining and low estrogen and progesterone levels. Some women may also experience lower back pain, diarrhea, or nausea.

✧ Emotional: Feelings of introspection, low energy, and a need for rest and retreat. Many women report a desire to withdraw socially and focus inward during this phase, reflecting the body's need to conserve energy and reset.

Connecting to the Seasons & the Moon:

✧ Theme Season: Winter
- Winter is a season of dormancy and conservation. In nature, many animals hibernate, and plants go into a state of rest. Similarly, the menstruation phase calls for a period of rest and introspection. It is a time to slow down, conserve energy, and reflect. The body is cleansing itself, both physically by shedding the uterine lining and metaphorically by encouraging inward focus and self-reflection. This phase is about renewal and preparing for new growth, much like winter precedes the rebirth of spring.

✧ Moon: New Moon
- The New Moon symbolizes new beginnings and a clean slate. Just as the moon cycle starts afresh, menstruation is the beginning of a new menstrual cycle. This phase encourages setting intentions for the upcoming cycle and focusing on what you wish to cultivate in the coming weeks. The New Moon's energy is quiet and introspective, mirroring the low energy and reflective mood often experienced during menstruation. This alignment with the lunar cycle highlights the natural rhythm and cyclical nature of women's bodies, fostering a deeper connection with the universe and its patterns.

Understanding menstruation as a phase of renewal and reflection helps in embracing this time with compassion and self-care. It is an opportunity to honor the body's natural processes and the cyclical patterns that guide our lives. By aligning with the energy of winter and the New Moon, we can use this phase to rest, set intentions, and prepare for the energetic shifts that will follow in the later phases of the menstrual cycle.

FOLLICULAR PHASE: THEME INNER SPRING

Duration: Approximately 7-10 days
Days: Day 1 to Day 11-14 of the cycle

What hormonally is going on:

- ✧ Estrogen: Levels begin to rise, promoting the thickening of the endometrial lining. Estrogen is primarily produced by the developing ovarian follicles and plays a crucial role in preparing the body for a potential pregnancy.
- ✧ Follicle-Stimulating Hormone (FSH): Stimulates the growth of follicles in the ovaries. Each follicle contains an immature egg, and the rise in FSH helps these follicles to mature.

What are some physical and emotional responses you might experience:

- ✧ Physical: During this phase, many women experience increased energy, clearer skin, improved cognitive function, and enhanced physical stamina. The body feels revitalized, akin to the awakening that happens in nature during spring.
- ✧ Emotional: Feelings of optimism, creativity, and social engagement are prevalent. Many women feel more outgoing, motivated, and open to new experiences at this time. Rising estrogen has a positive effect on mood and overall sense of well-being.

Connecting to the Seasons & the Moon:

- ✧ Season: Spring
    - ♦ Spring is a season of growth, renewal, and new possibilities. Just as the earth awakens and blossoms after the dormancy of winter, the follicular phase represents a time of renewal and new beginnings in the menstrual cycle. This phase is marked by increased vitality,

creativity, and a sense of fresh potential. The body is preparing for the possibility of new life, similar to how spring fosters new growth in nature. This period encourages setting new goals, taking on new projects, and embracing change with enthusiasm and hope.

- Moon: Waxing Crescent
  - The Waxing Crescent Moon phase follows the New Moon and is a time of growth and building towards fullness. During this lunar phase, the moon is increasing in light, symbolizing the process of development and expansion. This aligns perfectly with the follicular phase, where the body is preparing for ovulation and potential conception. The Waxing Crescent Moon's energy supports setting intentions, making plans, and starting new ventures. It is a time of hope and forward momentum, reflecting the biological and emotional changes occurring in the body.

Understanding the follicular phase as a period of growth and renewal allows us to harness its energy for personal development and creativity. By aligning with the rhythms of spring and the Waxing Crescent Moon, we can make the most of this phase's vibrant and hopeful energy, setting the stage for the fruition and abundance that follows in the ovulation phase. This holistic perspective encourages a harmonious connection between our menstrual cycle, nature, and the cosmos, fostering a deeper appreciation for the natural cycles that influence our lives.

OVULATION: THEME INNER SUMMER

Duration: Approximately 24-48 hours
Days: Day 12-16 of the cycle

What hormonally is going on:

- Estrogen: Peaks just before ovulation, which enhances the sensitivity of the body and prepares the reproductive system for the possibility of conception.
- Luteinizing Hormone (LH): Surges to trigger the release of the mature egg from the ovary. This LH surge is the most significant hormonal change that prompts ovulation.
- Follicle-Stimulating Hormone (FSH): Also peaks, though not as sharply as LH, supporting the final maturation of the follicle.

What are some physical and emotional responses you might experience:

- Physical: Increased libido, heightened senses, clear and glowing skin, and higher energy levels. Many women feel more attractive and physically vibrant during this phase.
- Emotional: Feelings of confidence, assertiveness, and social connectivity are prominent. This is often a time when women feel their best physically and emotionally, exhibiting enhanced communication skills and a desire for social interaction.

Connecting to Seasons and Moon:

- Season: Summer
  - Summer is characterized by warmth, abundance, and peak energy. It is a time of growth, fruitfulness, and outward expression. Similarly, ovulation represents the peak of the menstrual cycle's reproductive potential, a time when the body is most fertile and energetic. The vibrancy and confidence felt during ovulation mirror the vitality of summer, making it an ideal time for social activities, creative projects, and expressing oneself fully.
- Moon: Full Moon
  - The Full Moon symbolizes peak energy, culmination, and fruition. Just as the moon is at its brightest and fullest, ovulation represents the peak of fertility and the culmination of the follicular phase's preparation. The Full Moon's energy is potent and dynamic, encouraging connection, celebration, and the manifestation of intentions set during the New Moon. This alignment highlights the peak reproductive potential, and the sense of completeness and empowerment felt during ovulation.

Understanding ovulation as the peak phase of the menstrual cycle allows us to harness its abundant energy and potential. By aligning with the rhythms of summer and the Full Moon, we can fully embrace the heightened vitality and social connectivity of this phase. This perspective encourages a harmonious connection between our menstrual cycle, the natural world, and the lunar cycle, fostering a deeper appreciation for the cyclical nature of our lives and bodies.

LUTEAL PHASE: THEME INNER AUTUMN

Duration: Approximately 10-16 days
Days: Day 15-28 of the cycle

What hormonally is going on:

✧ Progesterone: Levels rise, preparing the endometrial lining for the potential implantation of a fertilized egg. Progesterone is crucial for supporting a pregnancy in its early stages.
✧ Estrogen: Levels initially dip after ovulation, then rise again midway through the luteal phase before dropping if pregnancy does not occur. This secondary rise in estrogen supports the thickening of the endometrial lining.

What are some physical and emotional responses you might experience:

✧ Physical: Common symptoms include bloating, breast tenderness, fatigue, and changes in appetite. Some women may also experience headaches, acne, and digestive issues. These physical changes are due to the increased progesterone and the body's preparation for a potential pregnancy.
✧ Emotional: This phase can bring about mood swings, irritability, anxiety, and depressive symptoms, particularly for those with Premenstrual Dysphoric Disorder (PMDD). Emotional sensitivity, decreased motivation, and a need for self-care and introspection are also common.

Connecting to the Seasons and Moon:

✧ Season: Autumn
  • Autumn is a season of winding down, preparation for rest, and reflection. It marks the transition from the vibrancy of summer to the dormancy of winter. The luteal phase mirrors this seasonal change as the body transitions from the peak energy of ovulation to a state of preparation for potential rest (menstruation). This phase encourages slowing down, evaluating the past cycle, and preparing for renewal. It is a time for introspection, self-care, and nurturing oneself, just as nature prepares for the quiet of winter.

- ✧ Moon: Waning Crescent
  - ♦ The Waning Crescent Moon phase is characterized by a decrease in light, symbolizing a time of releasing, letting go, and introspection. It represents the final stage of the lunar cycle before the New Moon begins again. Similarly, the luteal phase is a time for letting go of the potential for pregnancy if fertilization has not occurred and preparing for the new cycle. The energy of the Waning Crescent Moon supports self-reflection, closure, and setting the stage for new intentions in the upcoming cycle.

By learning these connections between the menstrual cycle, seasonal changes, and lunar phases, we can foster a deeper relationship with our bodies and embrace each phase with greater awareness and compassion. This holistic perspective not only honors the scientific aspects of our biology but also integrates the spiritual and emotional dimensions of our experiences.

WHAT ARE ALL THESE HORMONES?

Your Hormonal Guide

Your menstrual cycle is regulated by a complex interaction of hormones, each playing a crucial role in its different phases. Here's an overview of the primary hormones, their functions, and how they contribute to the cycle:

- ✧ **Follicle-Stimulating Hormone (FSH):** Stimulates the growth of ovarian follicles in the follicular phase.
- ✧ **Luteinizing Hormone (LH):** Triggers ovulation and supports the formation of the corpus luteum.
- ✧ **Estrogen:** Thickens the uterine lining, supports ovulation, and works in harmony with progesterone.
- ✧ **Progesterone:** Prepares the uterine lining for implantation and peaks in the luteal phase.
- ✧ **Gonadotropin-Releasing Hormone (GnRH):** Signals the release of FSH and LH, regulating the entire cycle.
- ✧ **Testosterone**: Plays a subtle yet vital role in energy, strength, and libido.

Understanding our fascinating bodies, our hormones, and their interactions can help you navigate your cycle with greater clarity and awareness.

HORMONAL SHIFTS IN THE LUTEAL PHASE

Understanding the luteal phase is critical for sufferers with PMDD, but frankly, it is important to know for all who menstruate. Most likely, this is the time that everyone experiences PMS symptoms, but PMDD is a severe form of premenstrual syndrome characterized by intense emotional and physical symptoms that interfere with daily life. It is when both progesterone and estrogen peak and plunge during this time and when women who have this abnormal sensitivity to the normal fluctuations of these hormones feel it all.

EARLY DETECTION THROUGH AWARENESS: A GAME CHANGER

Understanding the phases and hormones of the menstrual cycle empowers women and AFAB individuals to recognize patterns in their symptoms and distinguish between typical premenstrual changes and signs of PMDD. While some mood fluctuations and physical symptoms are normal, extreme emotional distress, debilitating physical discomfort, and significant disruption to daily life are indicators that call for further attention.

By educating women on what to expect during each phase, we enable them to identify abnormal symptoms early on. Imagine a world where mothers share and tell their daughters the importance of understanding their menstrual cycles.

This awareness is vital for early detection, allowing for prompt intervention through lifestyle adjustments and natural or medical treatments. Recognizing these patterns enhances self-awareness and promotes proactive health management, ensuring women receive the support they need to maintain their well-being throughout their menstrual cycles.

BREAKING THE SILENCE

For centuries, women's health, especially regarding menstrual cycles, has been cloaked in silence and stigma. This emotional suppression and the lack of comprehensive education about our bodies have left many of us feeling isolated, unseen, unheard, and misunderstood. This cultural legacy impacts not only our individual health but also our homes, communities, and society as a whole.

From an early age, many of us were taught to hide our menstrual experiences and dismiss our feelings as mere "PMS." Have you ever considered how we as women are still whispering about our periods or being so discreet with our menstrual products when we are in public, as if we still have something to hide or be ashamed about. This kind of feeling, this emotional suppression, can create a disconnection from our own experiences and hold within us a sense of shame about natural biological processes.

Experiencing PMDD or severe menstrual-related symptoms often means suffering in silence, believing our pain is normal, or fearing we will not be taken seriously. This suppression not only affects our mental health but can also strain relationships and disrupt daily life. Our partners, family members, and colleagues might not fully understand the depth of our struggles, leading to feelings of isolation and misunderstanding.

THE CONSEQUENCES OF BEING UNDEREDUCATED

The lack of education about menstrual health is a significant barrier to early detection and effective management of menstrual disorders. Many of us are unaware of the separate phases of the menstrual cycle and the roles hormones play in our physical and emotional well-being. This knowledge gap means abnormal symptoms often go unrecognized and untreated.

Without proper education, we are less likely to seek medical advice or interventions, perpetuating a cycle of ignorance and neglect. Misdiagnosis or delayed diagnosis of conditions like PMDD can result in prolonged suffering and inadequate treatment. Educating ourselves about our bodies empowers us to advocate for our health, seek proper care, and make informed decisions about our treatment options.

THE RIPPLE EFFECT ON CULTURE AND SOCIETY

The impacts of emotional suppression and inadequate education extend beyond individual experiences, affecting our culture and society. In homes where menstrual health is not openly discussed, young girls grow up without the knowledge and support they need to navigate their menstrual cycles confidently. This perpetuates a cycle of silence and stigma that affects generations.

In the workplace, the lack of understanding about menstrual health can lead to discrimination and a lack of accommodations for those experiencing severe symptoms. This not only affects our professional lives but also perpetuates gender inequality.

On a broader societal level, the silence around women's health issues contributes to a lack of research and resources dedicated to understanding and treating menstrual disorders. This gap in knowledge and funding hampers the development of effective treatments and interventions, leaving many of us without the support we need.

By breaking this silence and educating ourselves and others about menstrual health, we can begin to change the narrative. We can foster a culture of openness and support that helps us and future generations. Let's take this step together, advocating for our health and well-being.

A CALL FOR CHANGE

Breaking the cycle of emotional suppression and lack of education requires a collective effort. By fostering open conversations about menstrual health and educating women about their bodies, we can empower them to take control of their health and well-being.

- ✧ Education: Comprehensive education about the menstrual cycle, hormonal changes, and menstrual disorders should be integrated into school curriculums and healthcare practices. Women should be encouraged to track their cycles, recognize patterns, and seek medical advice when necessary.
- ✧ Awareness: Raising awareness about the emotional and physical impacts of menstrual health can help destigmatize these experiences and promote understanding. Media campaigns, public health initiatives, and community programs can play a crucial role in this effort.
- ✧ Support: Creating supportive environments at home, work, and in healthcare settings can help women feel seen, heard, and validated. This includes providing accommodations in the workplace, offering mental health support, and ensuring access to proper medical care.

By embracing education and emotional awareness, we can transform how women's health is perceived and treated, leading to healthier individuals, stronger families, and a more compassionate society. This shift benefits women and enriches our collective cultural fabric, fostering a world where everyone can thrive.

BREAKING THE CYCLE OF MISDIAGNOSIS

Historically, women's health issues, especially those related to the menstrual cycle, have been misunderstood and under-researched. This has often led to a cycle of misdiagnosis and inadequate treatment. Many women experiencing severe menstrual symptoms are initially diagnosed with conditions like depression, which, while sharing some symptoms, require different treatment approaches.

Comprehensive menstrual cycle education can help break this cycle. When women understand the specific symptoms and triggers of their menstrual health issues, they are better equipped to advocate for themselves in medical settings. They can provide healthcare professionals with detailed accounts of their symptoms, leading to more accurate diagnoses and effective treatment plans.

EMPOWERING THROUGH EDUCATION

Beyond the medical benefits, menstrual cycle education empowers women and AFAB personally and professionally. Knowledge of their cycles allows women to predict and manage their symptoms proactively. For example, they can plan demanding tasks around their more energetic phases and allow for self-care during the luteal phase.

In the workplace, this awareness can foster a more supportive environment. Women can communicate their needs more effectively and advocate for policies that accommodate their health, such as flexible work schedules or access to mental health resources.

Menstrual cycle education also plays a vital role in building supportive communities. When women share their experiences and knowledge, they create a network of support that reduces feelings of isolation and shame. This community support is invaluable, offering encouragement, shared resources, and a collective voice advocating for better healthcare and workplace policies. Integrating menstrual cycle education into our schools, healthcare systems, and workplaces is not just a women's issue. It is imperative.

A FUTURE OF AWARENESS AND EMPOWERMENT

As we bring awareness to the importance of menstrual cycle education, we lay the foundation for a future where every woman can thrive. By detecting early signs and signals of menstrual disorders, we move towards a world where women can live in harmony with their cycles, fully embracing their potential and contributing to society without the burden of untreated and misunderstood health issues. This is not just about managing symptoms but about reclaiming our health, power, and identity.

A WORLD LOOK ON MENSTRUAL CYCLE EDUCATION

In many developed countries, menstrual cycle education is integrated into school curriculums, though the depth and comprehensiveness can vary. Nations like Sweden and the Netherlands are often recognized for their progressive sex education programs, which include detailed information on the menstrual cycle, hormonal changes, and reproductive health.

The Impact:

- ✧ Improved Health Outcomes: Women and girls in these countries typically have better access to healthcare services and products, enabling them to manage their menstrual health effectively.
- ✧ Reduced Stigma: Comprehensive education helps normalize menstruation, reduce stigma, and foster a supportive environment.
- ✧ Early Detection and Treatment: With better knowledge, women can identify and seek treatment for menstrual-related disorders early, improving overall health and productivity.

In many developing countries, menstrual cycle education is often insufficient or entirely absent due to cultural taboos, lack of resources, and limited access to education, creating a significant knowledge gap. This gap has profound consequences for girls and women:

Health Risks: Poor menstrual hygiene practices, resulting from inadequate education, increase the risk of infections and other health complications.

Stigma and Shame: Menstruation is often shrouded in secrecy and shame, leading to isolation and a lack of support.

Missed Opportunities: Many girls miss school during their periods due to a lack of facilities and sanitary products, negatively affecting their education and future opportunities

Delayed Diagnosis: Without proper understanding, symptoms of menstrual disorders may go unrecognized and untreated, severely affecting quality of life.

Cultural beliefs and practices play a significant role in how menstruation is perceived and managed. In some cultures, menstruation remains a taboo subject, leading to various restrictions and misconceptions that can severely hinder menstrual education and health:

Restrictions and Isolation: Menstruating women may be isolated or restricted from daily activities, affecting their social and emotional well-being.

Limited Discussion: Cultural taboos often prevent open discussions about menstrual health, perpetuating misinformation, and myths.

Barriers to Education: These norms can hinder girls from learning about their bodies, reducing their ability to manage their menstrual health effectively.

The intersection of inadequate education and cultural taboos deepens the challenges women face, making menstrual health an urgent issue in many parts of the world. Reflecting on the diverse global approaches to menstrual cycle education, it is clear that where you live profoundly affects your understanding and management of menstrual health. Growing up in a society that openly discusses and educates about menstrual health can equip you with the knowledge to support your well-being, seek initial treatment for any issues, and navigate life with confidence and support.

By advocating for comprehensive menstrual cycle education globally, we can help break the cycle of misdiagnosis and mistreatment. This is not just a health issue; it is about empowering women to understand and take control of their bodies, reducing stigma, and fostering a more inclusive and supportive society. As we continue to raise awareness and push for better education, we pave the way for a future where every woman can thrive, fully embracing her potential without the burden of untreated or misunderstood health issues. This journey towards awareness and empowerment is crucial for reclaiming our health, power, and identity.

THE GLOBAL IMPACT OF MENSTRUAL CYCLE EDUCATION

Investing in menstrual cycle education has significant economic benefits. Educated women are healthier and more productive, contributing positively to the economy. Reducing menstrual-related absenteeism in schools and workplaces can lead to better educational outcomes and increased workforce participation.

Globally, improving menstrual cycle education can lead to better health outcomes. Early detection and treatment of menstrual disorders like PMDD can prevent long-term health issues. Proper menstrual hygiene management reduces the risk of infections and other related health problems.

Menstrual cycle education is a critical part of gender equality. By normalizing menstruation and providing the necessary education and resources, we can break down barriers that prevent women from taking part fully in society. This includes reducing the stigma associated with menstruation, ensuring access to sanitary products, and promoting policies that support menstrual health in schools and workplaces.

A GLOBAL CALL TO ACTION

Addressing the disparities in menstrual cycle education requires a multi-faceted approach involving governments, communities, and individuals.

1. **Policy Development:** Governments must prioritize menstrual health education in school curriculums and provide funding for menstrual health programs.
2. **Community Engagement:** Community leaders and influencers can play a significant role in breaking down cultural taboos and promoting open discussions about menstruation.
3. **Access to Resources**: Ensuring access to sanitary products and healthcare services is essential for managing menstrual health effectively.
4. **Research and Advocacy:** Continued research into menstrual health and disorders like PMDD is crucial for developing effective treatments and interventions. Advocacy efforts can help raise awareness and drive policy changes.

Understanding the menstrual cycle is the foundation for recognizing and addressing more complex menstrual health issues, such as Premenstrual Dysphoric Disorder (PMDD). When girls, women, and AFAB are not adequately educated about their cycles, they are left vulnerable to confusion and anxiety over symptoms they may experience, often without realizing there is a deeper issue at play. PMDD, a severe form of PMS, goes beyond the typical discomforts of menstruation, manifesting in emotional and physical symptoms that disrupt daily life. Without foundational knowledge of the menstrual cycle, recognizing the signs of PMDD and receiving proper care can be delayed. In the next chapter, we will explore what PMDD is, its symptoms, and how it affects the lives of those who experience it, highlighting the crucial role menstrual education plays in early identification and treatment.

Disclaimer: I am not a medical professional, and the insights shared in this book are based on personal experiences and extensive research. This book is intended to provide educational information and should not be considered a substitute for professional medical advice, diagnosis, or treatment. If you are seeking deeper understanding and professional guidance on menstrual health, I highly recommend exploring the book Wild Power: Discover the Magic of Your Menstrual Cycle and Awaken the Feminine Path to Power by Alexandra Pope and Sjanie Hugo Wurlitzer, as well as considering the various programs offered by experts in this field. Always consult with a healthcare provider for any medical concerns or conditions.

Chapter THREE

UNDERSTANDING PMDD

> *"PMDD is not a life sentence; it is a call to uncover the depths of who you truly are. It's an invitation to heal, transform, and reclaim the power within you, one cycle at a time."*
> **- Rachel Lynn Fox**

For far too long, women have been told to simply "cope" with the discomfort and mood swings that come with PMS, as if it is an inevitable part of womanhood to endure quietly. The expectations placed upon us are clear: keep pushing through, maintain our responsibilities, and suppress any signs of struggle, regardless of the physical and emotional toll. Society has normalized the idea that we should grit our teeth through the pain and frustration, often dismissing the profound impact PMS can have on our lives. We are expected to carry on, fulfilling our roles at work, home, and in relationships, all while managing symptoms that are often brushed off as something we should just "get used to." But what happens when the symptoms become more than just an inconvenience when they take over our lives? It is time to question these expectations and look deeper at how severe PMS profoundly affects us and what options exist beyond mere endurance.

While both PMS (Premenstrual Syndrome) and PMDD (Premenstrual Dysphoric Disorder) occur in the luteal phase of the menstrual cycle and share some common symptoms, there are critical differences between the two conditions in terms of severity, impact, and treatment approaches. It is essential to distinguish between PMS and PMDD to provide proper support and management strategies for those affected.

Premenstrual Syndrome (PMS) is a common condition affecting up to 75% of women and AFAB of reproductive age. PMS includes a wide range of physical and emotional symptoms, such as bloating, breast tenderness, fatigue, mood swings, irritability, and mild depression. These symptoms typically do not significantly interfere with daily functioning. While they can be uncomfortable and inconvenient, most women manage to continue with their usual activities and responsibilities.

In contrast, Premenstrual Dysphoric Disorder (PMDD) is a much more severe condition, affecting 3-8% of women and AFAB of reproductive age. PMDD includes extreme emotional and physical symptoms that can significantly disrupt daily life. Symptoms such as severe mood swings, intense depression, overwhelming anxiety, uncontrollable anger, and a heightened sensitivity to rejection are common in PMDD. These symptoms are not just inconvenient; they are debilitating, often causing profound distress and impairment in personal, social, and occupational functioning.

For those experiencing PMDD, the cyclical nature of the condition means that these severe symptoms occur predictably each month, typically during the luteal phase and resolving within a few days after menstruation begins. This regular recurrence of intense symptoms can make it feel like half of each month is consumed by emotional and physical turmoil, profoundly affecting the overall quality of life.

PMDD is a thief that lurks in the shadows of our monthly cycles, often unseen and unrecognized, but its impact is profound and deeply personal. For years, I struggled to understand why I felt like I was living an internal masked double life. On the surface, I was holding it all together, but inside, a storm was brewing every month, leaving me feeling isolated, misunderstood, and utterly alone. My journey through undiagnosed PMDD was marked by confusion, self-doubt, and a relentless search for answers that seemed always just out of reach. It literally never occurred to me that what I was experiencing was connected to my menstrual cycle.

Premenstrual Dysphoric Disorder does not discriminate. It does not matter how much money you make, where you live, or what your background is. It can affect anyone from any walk of life, turning our cycles into a rollercoaster of emotional and physical pain. While there are various premenstrual disorders, each with its unique challenges, my story and this book's focus on PMDD shares the lens through which I have viewed my world, and it is through understanding PMDD that I found my way to healing.

For too long, I was caught in a cycle of suffering that I could not name. The rage, the overwhelming sadness, the physical symptoms that seemed to come out of nowhere – all of it was dismissed as just a part of being a woman. But deep down, I knew it was more than that. It was only after countless doctor's visits, misdiagnoses, and late-night internet searches that I finally stumbled upon the term PMDD. It was a revelation, a moment of clarity that brought both relief and grief. Relief, because I finally had a name for my pain; grief, because of the years lost to this invisible enemy.

This chapter is dedicated to uncovering the truth about PMDD, shedding light on what it truly means to live with this condition. It is my hope that through sharing my journey with you that you will feel seen and validated, knowing that you are not alone in this fight. We will explore the nature of PMDD, understanding its symptoms, causes, and how it can be managed. Most importantly, we will begin the journey of reclaiming our lives from its grasp, finding hope and healing along these pages.

In the United States, about 1 in 12 women suffer from PMDD. The number typically includes those between the ages of 12 and 50, which accounts for about 25% of the total population, or approximately 83.5 million menstruators. So, 1 in 12 menstruators in the United States is approximately 7 million people.

The journey of living with undiagnosed PMDD can be incredibly challenging. Symptoms such as severe mood swings, depression, anxiety, and physical discomfort can dominate the lives of those affected, often leading to feelings of isolation and confusion. Many individuals wait an average of 12 years and consult multiple healthcare providers before receiving a correct diagnosis. My battle with PMDD was relentless, grueling, and exhausting, marked by a desperate search for answers. Each month, I was consumed by an overpowering sense that something was profoundly wrong, yet no one could name it. The severe mood swings, crippling depression, crying spells, and shame took a stranglehold on my life, leaving me spiraling into chaos and despair. This unending torment stripped away my sense of control, plunging me into deep isolation and a consuming desperation for understanding and relief. What has left me speechless and righteously angered still is that we all share the very same experience of going into our OBGYN's; we all fill out the same basic form, checking the box that we have a period while adding the date when we last had it. The form I filled out 30 years ago is the same form I fill out today. There has never been one form I have seen in a general doctor, an OBGYN, or a therapist's office that asks about PMS symptoms. No one is asking what we are emotionally or physically feeling or experiencing leading up to our period. NO ONE! How are we not asking these questions, especially if 75% of women experience PMS?!

Navigating life with PMDD often feels like being trapped in an unpredictable storm or like being stuck in a recurring nightmare. Each month, like clockwork, you may find yourself overwhelmed by a cascade of emotions and physical symptoms that can leave you feeling isolated and misunderstood. The suffering is profound and multifaceted, affecting every aspect of life. As someone who has walked this path, I understand the profound impact these symptoms can have on your daily life. From sudden and severe mood swings to deep feelings of depression and intense irritability, the experience of PMDD can be all-consuming. It is not just about feeling sad or anxious—it is a complete loss of control over one's emotions and body, creating a deep sense of hopelessness and isolation. Let's break down the suffering and symptoms that recur month after month, painting a vivid picture of this relentless cycle:

Here is the list of PMDD symptoms:

1. **Mood / Emotional Changes**: Sudden and severe mood changes, including periods of uncontrollable crying.
2. **Irritability or Anger**: Heightened sensitivity and easily triggered anger, often leading to conflicts with others.
3. **Depression:** Deep feelings of sadness, hopelessness, and worthlessness, sometimes accompanied by suicidal thoughts.
4. **Anxiety:** Intense feelings of tension, nervousness, and unease.
5. **Sensitivity to Rejection:** Drastic emotional pain or response from perceived or actual rejection, criticism, or abandonment.
6. **Decreased Interest in Activities**: Loss of interest in hobbies, social activities, and relationships.

7. **Difficulty Concentrating**: Problems with focus, memory, and decision-making.
8. **Fatigue:** Persistent tiredness and lack of energy despite adequate rest.
9. **Appetite Changes**: Overeating or specific food cravings, often for high-carbohydrate or sugary foods.
10. **Sleep Problems:** Insomnia or excessive sleeping, affecting daily routines and overall well-being.
11. **Feeling Overwhelmed or Out of Control**: Sensations of being unable to manage daily responsibilities and emotions.
12. **Physical Symptoms**: Breast tenderness and soreness, bloating, constipation, headaches, joint or muscle pain.

So, What Causes PMDD?

Understanding the causes of Premenstrual Dysphoric Disorder invites us to explore a complex interplay between traditional medical perspectives and holistic approaches. PMDD is not a hormonal imbalance disorder. PMDD is attributed to an abnormal sensitivity to the natural hormonal changes that occur during the menstrual cycle, particularly the fluctuations in estrogen and progesterone levels. This hormonal sensitivity is believed to affect neurotransmitter systems in the brain, especially serotonin, leading to the severe emotional and physical symptoms experienced by those with PMDD. Genetics, neurotransmitter imbalances, and environmental factors are all thought to contribute to this heightened sensitivity.

However, holistic views broaden the conversation by considering the whole person—mind, body, and spirit. This perspective suggests that unresolved emotional issues, trauma, nutritional deficiencies, gut health, lifestyle factors, and environmental toxins play significant roles in the manifestation of PMDD.

By integrating these traditional and holistic perspectives, we can develop a more comprehensive understanding of PMDD and create more effective, personalized treatment plans that address both the symptoms and their underlying causes.

COMMON VIEWS ON THE CAUSES OF PMDD

PMDD is understood to be caused by an abnormal response to the normal hormonal changes that occur during the menstrual cycle. Specifically, research shows that individuals with PMDD have heightened sensitivity to the fluctuations of estrogen and progesterone, which can affect the brain's neurotransmitter systems, particularly serotonin. This hormonal sensitivity can lead to severe mood disturbances and other symptoms associated with PMDD.

Here are the commonly shared views on what causes PMDD:

1. **Hormonal Sensitivity:** PMDD is considered to be caused by an abnormal reaction to normal hormonal changes during the menstrual cycle, particularly the fluctuations in estrogen and progesterone levels. Research suggests that women with PMDD are more sensitive to these hormonal changes, which affect neurotransmitter activity in the brain, especially serotonin.

2. **Serotonin Involvement:** Serotonin, a key neurotransmitter that regulates mood, sleep, and appetite, is believed to play a significant role in PMDD. The hormonal fluctuations can alter serotonin levels or its function in the brain, leading to the emotional and physical symptoms associated with PMDD.

3. **Histamine:** Histamine can influence the brain's neurotransmitters, like serotonin, which are linked to mood regulation. Estrogen increases histamine release and decreases the enzyme that breaks down histamine. During the luteal phase of the menstrual cycle, when estrogen levels fluctuate, this can lead to elevated histamine levels, potentially contributing to PMDD symptoms like mood swings, anxiety, irritability, and headaches.

4. **Genetic Factors:** Studies show a potential genetic component to PMDD, with certain genetic variations making some individuals more susceptible to the condition. This predisposition can affect how the body processes hormones and neurotransmitters.

5. **Psychosocial Factors**: While the primary cause of PMDD is biological, psychosocial factors such as stress, traumatic experiences, and pre-existing mental health conditions like anxiety or depression can exacerbate the symptoms. These factors do not cause PMDD but can influence its severity and how it manifests in different individuals.

6. **Environmental Triggers:** Certain lifestyle factors, including diet, lack of exercise, and substance use (like alcohol and nicotine), can worsen PMDD symptoms. These environmental triggers interact with hormonal and neurotransmitter changes to affect mood and physical well-being.

PMDD FROM A HOLISTIC PERSPECTIVE

From a holistic viewpoint, PMDD manifests deeper imbalances within the body and mind. Holistic approaches consider the interconnectedness of physical, emotional, and spiritual health, emphasizing the need to address underlying causes rather than just managing symptoms.

Emotional and Psychological Stress: Chronic stress, unresolved trauma, and emotional repression are believed to contribute to hormonal sensitivities and PMDD symptoms.

Nutritional Deficiencies: Inadequate intake of essential nutrients, such as magnesium, vitamin B6, and omega-3 fatty acids, can affect hormonal balance and neurotransmitter function.

Gut Health: The gut-brain axis plays a significant role in mood regulation. Imbalances in gut flora and digestive health can contribute to PMDD symptoms.

Lifestyle and Environmental Toxins: Exposure to environmental toxins and endocrine disruptors found in plastics, pesticides, and processed foods can interfere with hormone function. Detoxification and reducing exposure to these substances are common recommendations in holistic treatment plans.

Energetic Imbalances: Holistic medicine views the body as an energy system. Imbalances in energy flow, as understood in practices like acupuncture and Reiki, can manifest as physical and emotional symptoms.

By integrating both traditional and modern medicine with holistic methods, we can offer a comprehensive approach to understanding and managing PMDD. This approach aims not only to alleviate symptoms but also to address the root causes, ultimately restoring balance and harmony to the body, mind, and spirit.

TREATMENT OPTIONS

Traditional methods of managing PMDD symptoms have undoubtedly served their purpose over time, offering many women much-needed relief in the face of overwhelming physical and emotional distress. From lifestyle changes to medical interventions like antidepressants and birth control, these approaches have provided comfort and stability to those suffering, often saving lives when the weight of the disorder becomes unbearable. These treatments have been vital in helping women navigate the unpredictability of PMDD. For many, these methods have been lifelines, offering a sense of control and hope amidst the storm. Yet, as we continue to learn more about this disorder, there is space to explore innovative approaches and build upon the foundation that traditional treatments have laid.

Traditional medical approaches to managing PMDD encompass a spectrum of treatments aimed at alleviating symptoms and improving the quality of life for those affected. Initial recommendations often involve lifestyle modifications such as dietary changes, regular exercise, and stress management techniques. When lifestyle adjustments are insufficient, pharmacological interventions, including medications, SSRIs, and hormonal therapies, are commonly prescribed to stabilize mood and hormone fluctuations. For severe, treatment-resistant cases, surgical options like hysterectomy with bilateral oophorectomy may be considered as a last resort, though this approach carries significant risks, including induced menopause and potential long-term consequences. These diverse treatments reflect the complexity of PMDD and the importance of individualized care in addressing its multifaceted impact.

While traditional medical treatments for PMDD, such as antidepressants, hormonal therapies, and lifestyle changes, remain common, a growing number of individuals are turning to holistic approaches to manage and alleviate symptoms. This shift highlights a desire to address the root causes of PMDD through a comprehensive approach that considers the whole person—mind, body, and spirit. Recent statistics from the National Center for Complementary and Integrative Health (NCCIH) reveal a 20% increase in the use of complementary and alternative medicine over the past decade, underscoring the rising popularity of holistic care for PMDD and other chronic conditions. For many, traditional treatments come with significant challenges, including burdensome side effects and the overwhelming process of navigating complex medical regimens. These factors often drive individuals to explore holistic options, which aim to provide relief without compounding their struggles. Holistic care offers a personalized and empowering pathway to healing, resonating deeply with those seeking to reclaim their well-being on every level.

Holistic approaches to managing PMDD offer a comprehensive pathway to improved well-being by addressing the condition's physical, emotional, and spiritual dimensions. A balanced diet rich in whole foods and supplements like magnesium, calcium, and omega-3 fatty acids supports hormonal balance and reduces inflammation. Herbal remedies, including chaste berry and evening primrose oil, provide natural symptom relief. Mind-body practices such as yoga, meditation, reiki, and acupuncture foster emotional and physical harmony, while regular exercise boosts mood and reduces stress. Stress management techniques, including CBT and relaxation practices, alongside maintaining quality sleep, further aid symptom control. Emerging modalities like Rapid Transformational Therapy, functional medicine, and guided psychedelic journeys delve into the root causes, offering transformative healing potential. Aromatherapy, essential oils, and community support groups provide added layers of emotional support and relaxation. By tailoring these methods to individual needs, individuals can navigate their unique PMDD journey with hope and empowerment, embracing personalized solutions for lasting relief.

THE IMPACT OF PMDD: LIVING WITH THE MONSTER WITHIN

Living with PMDD is an intensely personal and deeply challenging journey, one that reshapes the very fabric of your daily existence. For those of us who endure this condition, it is not just a series of symptoms but a profound and often harrowing experience that changes every aspect of life. Imagine waking up each day feeling like a shadow of your true self, consumed by an emotional and physical storm that wreaks havoc on your mind and body. The severe mood swings, paralyzing anxiety, and deep depression become relentless companions, leaving you grappling with a sense of isolation and despair. Every month, it feels as though a powerful force within you takes over, dictating your thoughts and actions, making you a stranger to yourself and those around you. The impact is far-reaching, disrupting relationships, work, and your overall quality of life. Yet, within this struggle, there is a resilient spirit that seeks understanding and relief, yearning to reclaim control and find harmony amidst the chaos. This is the reality of living with PMDD, a journey of navigating through the darkest storms to find moments of light and hope.

Women with PMDD describe it as feeling like a shadow of their true selves, consumed by an emotional and physical storm that wreaks havoc on their lives. Common descriptions include:

"I'm only a shell of a person" - During the luteal phase, the intense symptoms can strip away one's sense of self, leaving behind a hollow, unrecognizable version of who they truly are.

"Living like there is a monster or demon inside of me" - The emotional volatility and severe mood swings can feel like an uncontrollable force within, leading to behaviors and feelings that are foreign and frightening.

"PMS on steroids" - While PMS is uncomfortable, PMDD is overwhelmingly intense, amplifying every symptom to a debilitating degree.

"Only living half of a life" - The cyclical nature of PMDD means that women often experience relief only for part of the month, with the other half dominated by the disorder, effectively cutting their lives in half.

"A Jekyll and Hyde existence" - The dramatic personality shifts make it feel like you are two different people, one calm and the other unrecognizable.

"A monthly masquerade party" - Hiding the severity of symptoms from others, putting on a brave face while internally struggling.

"A Hijacked life" - Feeling like your life is no longer your own, constantly disrupted by the overpowering effects of PMDD.

I understood all of these. My life was marked by a relentless cycle of emotional and physical turmoil. Imagine feeling like a shadow of your true self, consumed by a storm that wreaks havoc on your life, only to bleed and momentarily feel like yourself again. Yet, even in those fleeting moments of clarity and relief, a dark cloud looms overhead. The anticipation of impending doom casts a shadow over the good weeks, knowing that in just a week or two, you will be swept away by the tide of PMDD once more. This sense of never being totally free from its grip, always bracing for the next wave, is a constant and exhausting battle that defines the lives of those living with PMDD.

Imagine this horrible experience that repeats itself every month, a cycle of emotional and physical turbulence that begins after ovulation and extends until menstruation. This is the experience of living with PMDD, a condition that paints the luteal phase of the menstrual cycle with shadows of intense symptoms lasting one to two weeks. As soon as the relief of menstruation is felt, the cycle starts anew, a relentless loop that the average woman endures about 450 times over her lifetime, equating to nearly 30 years of potential PMDD impact.

The truth is, looking back on my own experience, it often brings me to tears now. I lived half of my menstruating life in deep emotional pain.

There truly is grief with PMDD because you know you are only living half the life that you have been given.

PMDD'S DEVASTATING IMPACT

Living with PMDD is like navigating a storm that affects every area of life, eroding self-esteem and mental health. The emotional waves bring about profound feelings of shame, guilt, and inadequacy, chipping away at self-confidence and self-worth. It is not just about mood swings; it is about a deeper, more persistent struggle that can open the door to other mental health conditions like depression and anxiety.

PROFESSIONAL BATTLES

Navigating the professional world while dealing with PMDD is like walking a tightrope during a storm. The workplace demands consistency, focus, and productivity, but PMDD can severely undermine these expectations, leading to a cascade of challenges that affect every aspect of one's career.

PMDD often brings with it cognitive impairments such as difficulty concentrating, memory issues, and mental fog. These symptoms can make even routine tasks feel insurmountable. Deadlines loom larger, and the ability to stay organized and efficient wanes. This decline in cognitive function not only diminishes productivity but also undermines confidence. What once was easy becomes a struggle, leaving the individual feeling inadequate and frustrated.

The impact of cognitive impairments is highly felt in job performance. Tasks take longer to complete, mistakes become more frequent, and the overall quality of work may suffer. This dip in productivity is not just noticeable to the individual but also to colleagues and supervisors. The pressure to maintain a high standard of work despite PMDD symptoms can be overwhelming, leading to a vicious cycle of stress and deteriorating performance.

The debilitating symptoms of PMDD can cause frequent absences from work. Severe pain, extreme fatigue, and intense emotional distress can make it impossible to function, let alone perform job duties effectively. These absences, whether due to sick days or the need to leave work early, can jeopardize job security. Employers may perceive the frequent time off as a lack of reliability, potentially affecting career advancement opportunities.

The emotional volatility associated with PMDD can spill over into workplace relationships. Irritability and mood swings may cause friction with colleagues and supervisors. Misunderstandings and conflicts can arise, creating a tense and uncomfortable work environment. The individual with PMDD might feel alienated and unsupported, while coworkers may be unsure how to offer help or may feel the need to distance themselves to avoid conflict.

MARRIAGE AND PARTNERSHIPS BURDENED

PMDD weaves its way into the fabric of intimate relationships, often causing significant disruptions and emotional turmoil. The cyclical nature of the disorder means that every month brings a new wave of challenges that can lead to communication breakdowns and growing emotional distance.

The emotional volatility of PMDD can make effective communication challenging. Partners may find themselves on edge, unsure of how to approach conversations without triggering an emotional response. Simple misunderstandings can escalate into major conflicts fueled by the heightened sensitivity and irritability that PMDD brings. The unpredictability of mood swings can make it difficult to keep a consistent and open line of communication, leading to feelings of confusion and helplessness on both sides.

As communication falters, emotional distance often follows. Partners may struggle to understand the cyclical nature of PMDD, finding it hard to separate the person they love from the symptoms of the disorder. This lack of understanding can lead to feelings of isolation for both partners. The one with PMDD may feel misunderstood and unsupported, while the other may feel pushed away and unable to help. This emotional chasm can widen with each cycle, eroding the foundation of the relationship.

The physical and emotional symptoms of PMDD can cast a shadow over sexual intimacy. The fatigue, pain, and emotional distress that go with the disorder can diminish the desire for physical closeness. When intimacy does occur, it may be tinged with anxiety and self-consciousness, further straining the relationship. Partners may feel rejected or confused, not realizing that the decline in sexual activity is linked to the overwhelming symptoms of PMDD rather than a lack of desire or affection.

The persistent nature of PMDD can lead to shared frustration and resentment. The partner without PMDD may feel burdened by the constant emotional care needed, while the person with PMDD may feel guilty for the strain their condition places on the relationship. Over time, these unaddressed feelings can build up, creating a cycle of resentment that mirrors the cycle of PMDD symptoms.

For me, being in a relationship that already felt fragile at times, especially while we were dating in New York City, brought out a lot of vulnerability. My insecurities and trust issues would often take over, leading me to question his intentions constantly. I found myself doubting his loyalty, wondering if he was cheating or hiding something, even when there was no real reason to. It was like my fears and anxieties were always lingering, making it hard to fully trust.

Then, without warning, a surge of heightened sensitivity would hit; even a small, seemingly harmless comment would cut deeply. It wasn't just about the words; it was about the place they hit inside of me. One offhand remark, maybe something about the way I handled a situation or how I did something, felt like confirmation of my deepest fears—that I am failing, that I am not enough, or that I am too much to handle.

At that moment, it is like the words would take on a life of their own, magnifying my insecurities. What might have been said casually, or even with good intentions, distorts into something much bigger—a rejection of who I am. It is as if the comment is confirming all the inner turmoil, I had been trying so hard to keep hidden. The pain is immediate, sharp, and visceral. And suddenly, I am not just reacting to the present moment but to all the times I felt unworthy or unloved.

This sensitivity can create a wall between you and your partner. You may start to question everything—wondering if they really see you or if they are just tolerating you. It becomes hard to trust their love when you are struggling to love yourself. The rejection feels personal, even though deep down, you know it might not be intended that way. But in that instant, it is hard to separate the truth from the distortion that PMDD creates, and it can leave you feeling isolated in a relationship that is supposed to be your safe haven.

And that is why navigating the storm of PMDD requires patience, understanding, and open communication. Partners must work together to develop coping strategies and support systems. Education about PMDD can help demystify the condition, allowing both partners to approach it with empathy and compassion. Couples therapy or support groups can provide a safe space to express feelings and learn new ways to connect.

Despite the challenges, many couples find that facing PMDD together strengthens their relationship. By acknowledging the impact of PMDD and actively working to support each other, partners can create a deeper bond and a more resilient partnership. Understanding that PMDD is a shared journey can transform the experience from one of isolation and frustration to one of mutual support and growth.

FRIENDSHIPS TESTED

Navigating friendships with PMDD feels like trying to hold onto sand slipping through your fingers. The fatigue, depression, and irritability that accompany PMDD often lead to social withdrawal, making it incredibly challenging to keep connections. Imagine feeling so exhausted and emotionally drained that the thought of socializing becomes overwhelming. This withdrawal is not a choice but a necessity for self-preservation, yet it can be easily misunderstood by friends.

When you are dealing with the heavy weight of PMDD, the idea of meeting friends for coffee or attending social gatherings can feel like climbing a mountain. The energy it takes to be present and engaged is often too much, leading to canceled plans and missed opportunities to connect. Over time, this pattern of withdrawal can lead to feelings of isolation, as friends might not understand the invisible battle you are fighting. They might perceive your absence as disinterest or neglect, not realizing that you are doing your best to cope with overwhelming symptoms.

Friends may not grasp the severity of PMDD, leading to misunderstandings. They might see your mood swings or irritability as personal attacks or signs of a deteriorating friendship. Explaining PMDD can be difficult, especially if friends have never heard of it or cannot relate to the experience. This lack of understanding can strain relationships, creating a sense of distance and frustration on both sides. Friends might feel hurt or confused by your behavior, while you might feel unsupported and misunderstood, deepening the emotional chasm.

Despite these challenges, it is possible to keep meaningful friendships. Open and honest communication is key. Sharing your experiences and educating friends about PMDD can foster empathy and support. Friends who genuinely care will make an effort to understand and accommodate your needs. They might offer to come over instead of going out or checking in with a simple text on days when you cannot muster the strength for a conversation. Building a supportive network of friends who understand your journey can provide a much-needed lifeline during difficult times.

FAMILY LIFE CHALLENGES

PMDD does not just affect the individual; it ripples through the entire family, affecting relationships and daily life in profound ways. The emotional and physical toll of PMDD can make parenting and keeping family harmony especially challenging, leading to feelings of guilt, frustration, and stress.

As a parent with PMDD, you might find yourself struggling to balance your own needs with the demands of your children. The intense symptoms can leave you feeling depleted, making it hard to be the patient, attentive parent you strive to be. Simple tasks like helping with homework or attending a school event can feel insurmountable on days when symptoms are at their peak. This can lead to feelings of guilt and inadequacy, as you wish you could do more but are limited by your condition.

The unpredictability and severity of PMDD symptoms can create a stressful home environment. Family members may not know what to expect, leading to tension and misunderstandings. Children might sense the emotional turbulence and feel confused or anxious, not understanding why mom seems different at certain times of the month. Partners might struggle to provide support while also managing their own feelings of helplessness and frustration. This constant state of flux can affect the overall well-being of the family, creating an atmosphere of stress and uncertainty.

Through my healing journey, I really had to step back and put myself in my daughter's shoes to see our home through their eyes and innocent hearts. Although I know I was trying to do my absolute best as a single mom, my heart breaks knowing that this was some of their experience, but it's the truth, it's real, it's raw…but this is what my undiagnosed PMDD symptoms and my emotional pain did in our home month after month.

Imagine being a child whose sense of stability is connected to their mother's presence, but each month, that stability seems to shift without warning. You hear the front door open after school, and your stomach tightens. Will she be the loving, playful mom today, or will she come through the door, barely holding it together? You can feel the tension before she even steps inside, bracing yourself for what is to come. You tiptoe around the house, trying not to make too much noise, avoiding eye contact just in case something small sets her off. The air feels thick like you are walking on eggshells, and you learn quickly how to be quiet, how to avoid, and how to suppress your own needs to keep the peace.

At times, you find yourself confused. Why was she so patient with you yesterday but now does not seem to have any tolerance for even a simple question? You start to feel like maybe it's you. Maybe you're the reason for the change, deep down, you pray it is not the truth.

Leading up to her coming home from work becomes a waiting game. Your anxiety builds as you try to read the mood the minute she walks in. It is exhausting trying to figure out how to be the child she needs right now while never really knowing what that is. You love her so much, but sometimes, it feels like you are carrying the weight of the entire family on your small shoulders.

That kind of uncertainty, where love and fear collide, shapes your sense of safety in ways that are hard to explain. As a child, you just want your mom to be the steady anchor she once was. But with PMDD in the picture, even the most secure bonds feel fragile, and every moment feels like a balancing act—one that leaves you both yearning for connection and fearful of the next unpredictable wave.

Looking back, I can see that our home felt like a battleground for a few days each month, as if I were fighting fires I did not know how to put out. I was consumed by guilt, shame, and grief, knowing those were days I could never get back, a time that I would never have again. Offering myself love, understanding, and forgiveness was incredibly difficult. But it soon became crystal clear, because the life of my family truly depended on it, I had to take responsibility for my own responses, behaviors, and emotions; I had to take ownership of my own healing—for them and for me. I had to get better, for their sake and my own, and reclaim the life we deserved.

This is why having PMDD requires open communication and educating our families. Helping family members understand the nature of PMDD can foster empathy and patience. Explaining that PMDD is a severe and chronic health condition, not a choice or a reflection of your feelings towards them, can help alleviate some of the misunderstandings. Family therapy or support groups can provide a safe space for family members to express feelings and develop coping strategies together.

Additionally, setting realistic expectations and creating a supportive home environment can make a significant difference. This might include delegating tasks on difficult days, tracking your cycle as a family, setting up a routine that accommodates your needs, and prioritizing self-care to manage symptoms more effectively. By working together, families can create a resilient support system that helps mitigate the impact of PMDD, fostering a sense of unity and understanding.

The impact of PMDD is far-reaching, affecting every aspect of a woman's life, from her sense of self and mental health to her relationships and professional aspirations. Understanding the profound challenges faced by women with PMDD is crucial for providing the support and compassion needed to navigate this debilitating condition. By acknowledging the reality of living with PMDD and striving for comprehensive and empathetic care, we can help those affected reclaim their lives and find balance and peace amidst the storm and chaos.

THE STRUGGLE FOR RECOGNITION

For years, PMDD loomed in the background of countless women's lives, often misunderstood and dismissed as an extreme form of PMS. The path to its recognition in the DSM-5 was driven by the persistent advocacy of those living with its debilitating symptoms, alongside the efforts of mental health professionals and dedicated researchers. This collaborative determination led to a significant milestone in 2013 when PMDD was officially classified as a distinct mental health disorder in the fifth edition of the Diagnostic and Statistical Manual of Mental Disorders (DSM-5).

The DSM-5 (Diagnostic and Statistical Manual of Mental Disorders, 5th Edition) is a comprehensive guide published by the American Psychiatric Association used by mental health professionals to diagnose and classify mental health conditions. It provides standardized criteria for diagnosing mental disorders, including descriptions of symptoms, and is widely used in clinical, research, and educational settings to ensure consistency and accuracy in diagnosing mental health conditions.

This inclusion marked a pivotal moment. It was the result of years of rigorous scientific research that distinguished PMDD's unique symptoms and severe impact from other mood disorders and PMS. Advocacy groups tirelessly campaigned to raise awareness, emphasizing the urgent need for formal recognition and better treatment options. Panels of experts meticulously reviewed clinical evidence, reaching a consensus on the diagnostic criteria that would finally acknowledge PMDD as a serious condition requiring specific interventions.

The DSM-5 recognition brought a wave of hope and validation to those affected by PMDD. It helped better diagnosis, increased awareness, and led to more effective treatment options. It was a significant leap forward in understanding the disorder, but the journey was far from over.

One of the most alarming aspects of PMDD is its strong association with suicidal thoughts and behaviors. Imagine living with a condition where 72% of individuals report experiencing suicidal thoughts at some point in their lives—a stark contrast to the 10% in the general population. Nearly half of those with PMDD have made plans for suicide, and 34% have attempted it. These figures are not just numbers; they represent lives teetering on the brink, highlighting the urgent need for more research, early detection, and more education.

These statistics underscore a critical need for clinical guidelines that include regular screenings for suicide risk among individuals diagnosed with PMDD. Early intervention and proper mental health support are paramount to preventing these devastating outcomes. The recognition of PMDD in the DSM-5 is just one step in a longer journey toward comprehensive care and understanding.

GLOBAL IMPACT AND THE PATH FORWARD

The global burden of PMDD is staggering. With a prevalence of 5.5% among women and AFAB individuals of reproductive age, millions worldwide grapple with this condition. For instance, approximately 7 million women in the United States, 824,000 in the United Kingdom, 475,000 in Canada, and 20 million in India live with PMDD. Despite its prevalence, PMDD remains underdiagnosed and misunderstood, leading to significant personal, professional, and social challenges.

A GLIMMER OF HOPE

By recognizing the profound impact of PMDD and advocating for better diagnostic criteria and treatment options, we can improve the quality of life for those affected. This includes exploring both traditional treatments and innovative approaches in neuroscience and neuroplasticity. The journey toward understanding and managing PMDD is ongoing, but with continued advocacy, research, and empathy, we can offer hope and support to those navigating this challenging condition.

The story of PMDD's recognition in the DSM-5 and the urgent need to address its association with suicidal thoughts and behaviors is a testament to the power of advocacy and the importance of continued research and support. It is a journey that underscores the resilience of those affected and the critical need for a comprehensive approach to mental health care.

THE LONG AND WINDING ROAD TO DIAGNOSIS

The path to a PMDD diagnosis is often long, confusing, and emotionally taxing, marked by frequent misdiagnoses and fragmented care. Many individuals start by visiting general practitioners or gynecologists, who may misinterpret PMDD symptoms as generalized anxiety, depression, or hormonal imbalances, overlooking the cyclical nature of the condition. Specialists such as endocrinologists or mental health professionals often address isolated aspects of PMDD without treating its root causes, leading to partial or temporary relief. Frustrated by the lack of clear answers, many turn to self-diagnosis through online resources and support groups, often feeling isolated and misunderstood. The journey is further complicated by trial and error with treatments, ranging from medications with distressing side effects to lifestyle changes that may offer only limited relief. Emerging research into potential links between PMDD and other conditions, such as ADHD or autism, offers hope for improved understanding and diagnostic tools. Tracking your symptoms is a vital step in recognizing PMDD's patterns, and tools like the Stardust app provide a practical and empowering way to begin this process today. (I have also included a luteal phase symptom self-assessment tool at the end of this book.)

THE PATH FORWARD

By addressing the challenges of PMDD diagnosis requires a comprehensive approach focused on increasing awareness, improving diagnostic tools, and advancing research. Educating healthcare providers to recognize PMDD's unique patterns and distinguish it from other mood disorders is essential to reducing misdiagnoses and delays. Enhanced diagnostic protocols and ongoing research into comorbidities and targeted treatments are vital to offering better support and management. While the recognition of PMDD in the DSM-5 was a significant milestone, many individuals still face a long and difficult journey. By advocating for improved clinical practices and creating a more compassionate healthcare system, we can transform the PMDD experience from one of frustration to a pathway of hope and healing. We must do better.

To my daughters Naomi, Ella & my husband John:

There were days when I was a storm—

Unraveled, raw, and worn,

A shadow of the person you once knew,

But beneath it all, I was fighting to break through.

My heart was full of love, even still,

Though at times, the pain would spill.

Each wave of rage, each tear I cried,

It wasn't who I was but where I hurt inside.

You held me close when I fell apart,

Saw the cracks yet loved my heart.

In your embrace, I found my way,

Through darkest nights and heavy days.

Please forgive me when I couldn't speak,

The times I crumbled, feeling lost and weak.

Know that behind the shifting tide,

I was still there, trying to survive.

Your love was the light that softened me

Through undiagnosed and diagnosed PMDD.

And though I struggled, I always knew,

It was your love, your strength, that carried me through.

Thank you for your precious love. I love you dearly.

Chapter FOUR

BECOMING UNSTUCK IN AN ENDLESS CYCLE OF CHAOS

> *"The less you hold, the more your hands are open to what's here, unexpected, transformative. In every moment is the possibility for a new discovery, a radical undoing."*
> **— JAN FRAZIER**

Living with Premenstrual Dysphoric Disorder (PMDD) often feels like being trapped under a dark, oppressive cloud. Each month, the cycle repeats itself with relentless precision, bringing a storm of emotional and physical symptoms that can turn life into endless chaos. The impending gloom that accompanies PMDD can make even the simplest tasks seem insurmountable, leaving those affected feeling stuck in patterns of despair and helplessness.

I know this chapter is going to get deeply reflective, personal, and challenging, but you are here because something about this book has resonated with you and brought you to this moment right now. Trust your leading. It is crucial that we view our experiences for what they truly are rather than hiding in the shadows of our thoughts, emotions, and patterns. With an open heart and loving compassion, I pray these words land deeply within you, opening the portals of light that call to awaken you to the states and patterns that have controlled you. This journey is about shedding light on our truths and embracing the empowerment that comes from understanding and transformation.

The luteal phase, known as our "inner fall-autumn," occurs after ovulation and before menstruation in the menstrual cycle. During this time, hormones rise and fall, creating a shift that mirrors the season of autumn—a time of introspection, slowing down, and shedding what no longer serves us. It is from this lens we explore what PMDD is.

Just as the leaves begin to fall from the trees, the luteal phase encourages us to release emotions, patterns, and energies we have been carrying, particularly those we have been suppressing throughout the earlier parts of the cycle. This phase often brings heightened sensitivity, revealing truths about our unmet needs, unresolved emotions, and the parts of ourselves we may have been neglecting. It can be uncomfortable as these dark emotions rise to the surface, but this discomfort is a signal for reflection and transformation.

The invitation during the luteal phase is to embrace the message of wisdom of your body and mind. It's a time to truly honor your emotions, listen to your intuition, and create space for self-care and deeper self-reflection. Instead of pushing through and fighting it, we are being asked to slow down and explore the shadows within ourselves. This is the phase to nurture yourself, to go inward, and to prepare for the release and renewal that comes with menstruation—our "inner winter."

The luteal phase is an opportunity to integrate the lessons of your cycle, to let go of what no longer aligns with your highest self, and to embrace your inner truth. It is an invitation to heal, transform, and awaken.

Shifting into this new perspective, where we honor the call to slow down and release, can feel unsettling, especially when we are accustomed to pushing through or suppressing what comes up. The discomfort in this phase is not a punishment; it is a reflection of the deeper work waiting to be done. Often, this resistance keeps us stuck, clinging to old ways where we feel at the mercy of our emotions, our circumstances, and our bodies.

The difficulty lies in surrendering to this shift—moving away from the belief that we are powerless in the face of our cycle or that we must endure this phase in all its suffering. When we resist the invitation of the luteal phase, we stay trapped in old patterns, perpetuating cycles of pain and frustration. But when we allow ourselves to open to what is surfacing, we can move beyond what holds us back. This surrender becomes the key to moving from a place of victim to empowerment.

It is in this vulnerability, in acknowledging the emotions and unmet needs that arise, that we find our power to transform. By choosing to shift our perspective, we create space to release what no longer serves us and, instead, embrace healing, self-awareness, and the possibility of true growth. This is where the magic of the luteal phase lies—the opportunity to step out of the cycle of being stuck and step into something new.

This is not easy because, most likely, you have only viewed your experiences through the lens of being a victim of PMDD. I get it. That was me too. For so long, the intense emotional and physical symptoms have dictated your life, leading you to feel powerless and at the mercy of your condition. The cyclical nature of PMDD can create a sense of inevitability, where each month, you brace yourself for the onslaught, reinforcing feelings of helplessness and despair. It is natural to fall into patterns of casting blame, frustration, and withdrawal, believing that your suffering is unchangeable. However, recognizing these patterns is the first step towards reclaiming your power. By shifting your perspective, you can begin to see yourself not as a victim but as a resilient individual capable of navigating and transforming your experiences. This shift is pivotal in breaking free from the chains of victimhood and moving towards a place of empowerment and healing.

THE DARK CLOUD OF VICTIMHOOD CONSCIOUSNESS

A victim is someone who has suffered harm, injury, or loss due to circumstances beyond their control. In the context of emotional and mental well-being, a victim mentality or victim consciousness is a state of mind in which an individual perceives themselves as perpetually oppressed and powerless. This mindset is characterized by constant feelings of helplessness, blame, and resentment towards external factors or people. Individuals with a victim mentality often believe that they have no control over their lives and that their circumstances are dictated solely by others or by fate. This pervasive sense of powerlessness can lead to passive behavior, withdrawal, and a lack of initiative, trapping them in a cycle of negativity and self-fulfilling prophecies.

The relentless nature of PMDD can lead to a state of victimhood consciousness—a mindset where individuals feel trapped, powerless, and as though their lives are dictated by external circumstances beyond their control. In my years of taking part in PMDD Facebook groups and Reddit communities, I have seen an almost ingrained need to remain in a state of suffering. The very mention of hope or healing is often unwelcome, creating an environment where sharing positive experiences or breakthroughs is discouraged or outright rejected. While these support groups can provide a safe space for validation and understanding, they can sometimes become toxic to personal growth and healing. Forgive me if this observation feels offensive, but I offer it as an invitation to view the situation from a different perspective. I, along with my clients have shared posts or comments about our healing experiences and they are denied or removed from these groups, reflecting a broader resistance to acknowledging the possibility of recovery and transformation from PMDD.

SIGNS OF PMDD VICTIM CONSCIOUSNESS

Recognizing the signs of victim consciousness is the first step toward breaking free from its limiting grasp. This mindset can subtly infiltrate various aspects of one's life, creating a pervasive sense of helplessness and despair. Here are the key indicators that you or someone you know may be experiencing a state of victim consciousness:

1. **Constant Blame**: One of the clearest signs is a tendency to blame others or external circumstances for personal problems. This might involve blaming partners, family members, colleagues, or even fate for one's suffering and difficulties.
2. **Feelings of Powerlessness:** Individuals with a victim mentality often feel they have no control over their lives. They believe that their actions will not change their circumstances and that they are at the mercy of external forces.
3. **Negative Self-Talk:** Engaging in frequent negative self-talk is a hallmark of victim consciousness. Phrases like "I can't do anything right," "Why does this always happen to me?" and "I'm always unlucky" are common.
4. **Passive Behavior:** There is often a lack of initiative or passivity in decision-making. Instead of taking proactive steps to improve their situation, individuals may wait for others to intervene or for circumstances to change on their own.

5. **Dependence on External Validation:** Those in a victim mindset may seek constant validation and approval from others. Their sense of self-worth is often tied to how they are perceived by those around them.
6. **Avoidance of Responsibility:** Shunning personal responsibility for one's actions or life situation is another key sign. This avoidance can manifest as making excuses, deflecting accountability, or insisting that change is impossible.
7. **Resentment and Anger:** Harboring deep-seated resentment and anger towards people, life events, or society is common. This bitterness can poison relationships and hinder personal growth.
8. **Chronic Pessimism:** A persistent negative outlook on life, expecting the worst outcomes and seeing challenges as insurmountable obstacles, is a clear indicator. This pessimism reinforces the belief that one is destined to suffer.
9. **Isolation and Withdrawal:** Due to feelings of mistrust or fear of further hurt, individuals may withdraw from social interactions, leading to isolation. They may also avoid new experiences or opportunities due to fear of failure.
10. **Repetitive Patterns**: Experiencing the same negative outcomes repeatedly without recognizing the role one's mindset and actions play in perpetuating these patterns. This can create a sense of being stuck in a never-ending cycle.

Meet Sarah, a 32-year-old woman who has been struggling with PMDD for 10 years. Her condition has infiltrated various aspects of her life, creating a constant sense of helplessness and despair. Sarah's experiences illustrate the key indicators of victim consciousness.

Sarah often blames her partner, David, for not understanding her condition. She feels that if he were more supportive, her symptoms would be more manageable. She also blames her workplace for not accommodating her needs, and she often curses her fate for having to endure PMDD in the first place. This constant blame prevents her from taking any personal responsibility or looking for proactive solutions.

Every month, as her luteal phase approaches, Sarah feels a wave of powerlessness wash over her. She believes that no matter what she does, the debilitating symptoms will take over, and she has no control over her life during this time. This feeling of being at the mercy of her hormones makes her passive and reluctant to try new coping strategies.

Negative self-talk is a hallmark of victim consciousness and a barrier to empowerment. Sarah's internal dialogue is filled with negative self-talk. She often tells herself, "I can't do anything right," "Why does this always happen to me?" and "I'm always unlucky." As her luteal phase approaches, Sarah dreads the onset of symptoms, thinking, "Here comes Hell Week; this is going to be the worst luteal phase; I can feel it." These thoughts become a self-fulfilling prophecy, reinforcing her sense of inadequacy and failure.

When it comes to managing her PMDD, Sarah is often passive. Instead of seeking out new treatments or lifestyle changes that might help, she waits for her symptoms to subside on their own. She relies heavily on John to take over household responsibilities and avoids making decisions that could potentially improve her situation.

Sarah's self-worth is closely tied to how others perceive her. She constantly seeks validation from David, her friends, and her colleagues, needing their approval to feel good about herself. When she does not receive the validation she craves, her sense of worth plummets, reinforcing her victim mentality.

When her symptoms lead to conflicts or mistakes at work, Sarah avoids taking responsibility. She makes excuses, attributing her behavior entirely to her PMDD, and insists that there is nothing she can do to change the situation. This avoidance prevents her from learning and growing from her experiences.

Sarah harbors deep-seated resentment and anger towards her condition, her partner, and even herself. She feels bitter about her condition and often lashes out at David, blaming him for not being more empathetic. This bitterness strains her relationships and hinders her personal growth.

Sarah has a persistently negative outlook on life. She expects the worst outcomes and sees every challenge as an insurmountable obstacle. This chronic pessimism reinforces her belief that she is destined to suffer and that nothing will ever improve.

Due to her mistrust and fear of further hurt, Sarah withdraws from social interactions. She avoids seeing friends and taking part in activities she once enjoyed, leading to increased isolation. Her fear of failure keeps her from trying new things or pursuing opportunities that might bring joy or relief.

Sarah finds herself stuck in a cycle of repetitive negative outcomes. Each month, her symptoms lead to conflicts with David, mediocre performance at work, and a deepened sense of despair. She does not recognize how her mindset and actions perpetuate these patterns, feeling stuck in a never-ending cycle of suffering.

Sarah's story highlights the signs of victim consciousness that can accompany PMDD. Recognizing these patterns is the first step toward breaking free from their limiting grasp. By shifting her perspective and adopting proactive strategies, Sarah can begin to reclaim her power and move towards a life of empowerment and fulfillment. Is her experience landing with you?

BREAKING FREE FROM VICTIM CONSCIOUSNESS

Recognizing the signs of victim consciousness can be extremely difficult yet crucial. Overcoming this limiting mindset involves several steps, each essential for transitioning from a state of helplessness to one of empowerment.

SELF-AWARENESS

Becoming aware of one's thoughts and behaviors that contribute to a victim mindset is the foundational step. Self-awareness involves introspection and honest self-reflection to find patterns of thinking and behaving that perpetuate feelings of powerlessness. Keeping a journal or practicing mindfulness can help in observing these patterns without judgment, creating a space for understanding and change.

RESPONSIBILITY

Taking responsibility for one's actions and recognizing the power of choice is empowering. It means acknowledging that while external circumstances may be challenging, one's responses and attitudes are within their control. This shift from blaming external factors to taking ownership of one's life is transformative, fostering a sense of agency and possibility.

REFRAMING YOUR THOUGHTS

Challenging and reframing negative beliefs is essential for adopting a more empowered perspective. Cognitive-behavioral techniques can be helpful in identifying irrational or unhelpful thoughts and replacing them with more constructive ones. For instance, transforming "I can't handle this" into "I have faced challenges before and can find ways to cope" can significantly alter one's outlook and emotional response.

NEGATIVE SELF-TALK

Negative self-talk is a hallmark of victim consciousness and a barrier to empowerment. It involves recognizing and addressing the inner critic that perpetuates feelings of inadequacy and failure. Practicing self-compassion and affirmations can counteract negative self-talk. Instead of dreading the upcoming luteal phase with thoughts like, "Here comes Hell Week. This is going to be the worst luteal phase ever," Sarah can use affirming statements such as, "I am strong and capable of handling whatever comes my way," and "Each month, I learn more about managing my symptoms effectively." These positive affirmations help rewire the brain toward a more supportive self-dialogue and foster a sense of resilience.

SEEKING SUPPORT

Engaging with supportive communities, therapists, or coaches who can provide guidance and encouragement is vital. These support systems offer validation, new perspectives, and practical advice, making the journey less isolating. Therapy, especially modalities like trauma-focused Cognitive Behavioral Therapy, can be particularly effective in addressing deep-seated beliefs and emotional wounds.

BUILDING RESILIENCE

Developing resilience through practices such as mindfulness, self-compassion, and proactive problem-solving strengthens one's ability to cope with stress and adversity. Mindfulness helps one stay present and reduce anxiety about future challenges, while self-compassion fosters a kinder relationship with oneself. Proactive problem-solving involves finding issues and taking steps to address them rather than being overwhelmed by them.

EMPOWERMENT

Focusing on small, actionable steps to regain a sense of control and build confidence is crucial. Setting and achieving small goals creates momentum and proves that change is possible. Celebrating these small victories reinforces a sense of competence and empowerment, encouraging further progress.

Transitioning out of a victim mentality can be a difficult, gradual process that requires patience and dedication. However, by recognizing these signs and committing to change, it is possible to break free from the confines of victimhood and move towards a life of empowerment and fulfillment. Each step—self-awareness, taking responsibility, reframing thoughts, addressing negative self-talk, seeking support, building resilience, and focusing on empowerment—contributes to a more empowered and fulfilling life despite the challenges of PMDD.

Take a moment for self-reflection. The journey inward helps us understand our patterns and recognize where we might be giving away our power. Here are some questions to guide you:

1. In what areas of my life do I feel the most powerless, and why?

   _____

   _____

   _____

2. What traits of victimhood consciousness do I truthfully identify with

   _____

   _____

   _____

3. ?How do I react when faced with challenges or setbacks? Do I tend to blame external circumstances or others?

   _____

   _____

   _____

4. What stories do I tell myself about my life and experiences? Are they empowering or disempowering?

   _____

   _____

   _____

5. How often do I seek validation or approval from others to feel good about myself?

_____
_____
_____

6. What are my core beliefs about my ability to create change in my life

_____
_____
_____

7. ?How do I respond to criticism or feedback? Do I see it as an opportunity for growth or a personal attack?

_____
_____
_____

8. In what ways do I avoid taking responsibility for my actions and their consequences, typically during my luteal phase?

_____
_____
_____

9. How do I handle feelings of resentment or bitterness? Do I hold onto them or find ways to let them go?

_____
_____
_____

10. What steps can I take to shift from a victim mindset to one of empowerment and agency?

_____

_____

_____

11. How can I cultivate a greater sense of gratitude and appreciation for the positive aspects of my life?

_____

_____

_____

Reflecting on these questions can help illuminate areas where you may be operating from a place of victim consciousness. Awareness is the first step toward transformation and reclaiming your power.

When you begin to realize the cyclical nature of your emotions—the ones you once fiercely defended as righteous anger, justified by your bitterness, or guarded by your fear—you start to see that these defenses are just no longer serving you. What once felt like a form of protection, a way to shield yourself from deeper pain, has now become a burden. A burden that your body is telling you to put down. The stories you told yourself about your suffering, the way you clung to resentment, anger, or fears, were never meant to be carried forever.

And it is in this moment of awareness that transformation begins. Here, we start to tune into the wisdom of our luteal phase—our inner fall—and embrace the opportunity for deep self-reflection. What is your body trying to tell you? What messages lie within, urging you to listen and understand?

You might be starting to feel the weight of it all—years of emotional armor, built to survive, but now keeping you stuck. Your body begins to whisper what you have been ignoring: your body is tired. It is weary from fighting the same battles; it is exhausted from carrying the same scars, the same pain, over and over again. The anger that once fueled you now drains you. The bitterness that sharpened your perspective now clouds your ability to see clearly. The fear that kept you safe now keeps you from moving forward.

Your body is speaking louder than ever, sending signals of fatigue, tension, and heaviness. These are no longer just symptoms of PMDD or your cycle—they are the manifestations of emotional weight that you have been holding onto. You feel it in your bones, in the deep ache of your muscles, in the way your spirit feels exhausted before the day even begins.

This is the moment when you know something must shift. You can no longer carry the load because it is no longer aligned with how you want to live, how you want to feel and who you want to be. The defenses you built have served their purpose, but you are no longer in the same place you were when they were necessary. Now, they only hold you back, keeping you trapped in a loop of pain and exhaustion.

And now, it is in this space, this raw vulnerability of your truth, where the possibility for real change emerges. You are tired of the struggle, tired of fighting the same internal battles, and tired of living in a body that feels like a battlefield. Your body is asking for release, and your soul is ready for transformation. The realization that this cycle is no longer serving you marks the beginning of a new journey—a journey of letting go, embracing healing, and finally allowing yourself to step into a place of peace

Chapter Five

THE ROAD LESS TRAVELED

Two roads diverged in a yellow wood,
And sorry I could not travel both
And be one traveler, long I stood
And looked down one as far as I could
To where it bent in the undergrowth;

Then took the other, as just as fair,
And having perhaps the better claim,
Because it was grassy and wanted wear;
Though as for that the passing there

Had worn them really about the same,
And both that morning equally lay
In leaves no step had trodden black.
Oh, I kept the first for another day!
Yet knowing how way leads on to way,
I doubted if I should ever come back.

I shall be telling this with a sigh
Somewhere ages and ages hence:
Two roads diverged in a wood, and I—
I took the one less traveled by,
And that has made all the difference.
- Robert Frost

THE ROAD LESS TRAVELED: EMBRACING A NEW PATH FOR PMDD

I stood at a crossroads, much like the one Robert Frost described in his timeless poem. Two roads diverged before me: one well-trodden and familiar, the other less certain, shrouded in mystery. My journey with PMDD had brought me to this pivotal moment, exhausted from battling a relentless cycle of symptoms, searching for answers, and longing for relief.

The well-trodden path was one many before had taken. It promised quick fixes through medications, a band-aid solution that might alleviate symptoms but often came with a rocky road of side effects. It was the route most recommended, the one that seemed logical and endorsed by countless doctors and pharmaceutical companies. But after hitting dead end after dead end, I began to wonder: Is there really another approach? Is there truly a different road that leads to healing the root cause?

I did not know this alternative path existed. My upbringing and faith had convinced me that traditional medicine or divine intervention were my only options. But perhaps, in His infinite wisdom, God had developed a way many do not know of—one that does not involve filling the pockets of big pharma or relying solely on prescription drugs. Instead, it is a path that calls us individually to own our symptoms, our responses, behaviors, and our emotions by exploring them deeper through inner work and self-reflection.

EMBRACING THE JOURNEY OF OWNERSHIP

Here is the truth: our emotions, responses, and even those annoying triggers we stumble over—they are ours. They are not random occurrences or situations being thrown at us by the universe to dodge them, to drive us crazy, or to blame others. They are often very intimate parts of our story, connected to our past, and once this connects and resonates with you, you have now become that much more empowered. This can be a very influential moment in your life as you reclaim your personal power. It is about moving from asking, "Why is this happening to me?" to declaring, "What am I going to do about it?" This shift, my dear friends, is where true empowerment and real change begin.

Taking responsibility for your path means confronting the truth, even when it is one you would rather avoid. And believe me, I understand how hard that can be. After years of self-medicating, hiding, denying, and blaming others for most of my life, I know firsthand how challenging it is to finally face your experiences and claim them as your own for the first time.

It is acknowledging that you have been the victim in some chapters of your story and deciding you do not want to stay in that role. It is about looking at the person in the mirror and realizing that they have more strength and resilience than given credit for. And yes, it is about acknowledging that while we cannot control everything that happens to us, we can control how we respond.

Let's be clear: owning your journey is not about covering up the pain and pretending it is gone. It is about cultivating deep self-awareness, practicing radical honesty, embracing transparency, and reflecting with compassion. It is about diving into the depths of your emotions, understanding their origins, and gently guiding yourself through them on the path to true healing.

CHOOSING THE ROAD LESS TRAVELED

As we step into this chapter together, let's continue with a bit more curiosity. What if you stopped playing the blame game and stopped seeing yourself as just a character in someone else's story? How would that change your life? What would that feel like for you? Take a moment to really sit with these questions. They are big, and for many of you, it may be the first time you have considered them. Now, imagine stepping into your life as the author of your own story—owning every line, every paragraph, every chapter—the highs, the lows, and everything in between. And what if, by truly listening to the messages and cues your body is giving you, you realize it is time to finally let go of what has been holding you back?

This chapter is your invitation to a journey of ownership—a journey where you embrace the beautiful messiness of being human, learn to navigate your emotions with grace and courage, honor your body's messages, and discover the incredible strength that lies in vulnerability and forgiveness. It is time to take a deep breath, look within, and start walking this road of self-discovery. Trust me; the destination is worth every step.

Standing at this crossroads, I invite you to consider a new path. It is a path that may seem daunting, but it holds the promise of true healing and transformation. This journey is not about choosing an easy fix; it is about embracing the depth of your experiences and finding strength in your sensitivities and your vulnerabilities.

You see, our emotions, our triggers, and our responses are not just obstacles—they are gateways to deeper understanding and empowerment. By choosing to own our journey, we move from being passive recipients of our circumstances to active participants in our healing. It is about transforming our perspective from 'Why is this happening to me?' to 'How can I act and respond? This emphasizes a shift from feeling like a victim of circumstances to taking proactive steps toward solutions.

And let me be very clear on this, this road less traveled is not about rejecting traditional medicine or dismissing the value of medical interventions. Traditional medicine can be an answer for some, and there is no denying or shaming that. Traditional methods are helping countless sufferers experience relief, but this is about complementing those approaches though a different lens one with a profound commitment to inner work and self-discovery. It is about recognizing that true healing often involves looking inward, facing our fears, and cultivating a compassionate relationship with ourselves.

A NEW BEGINNING

As we move deeper, it is essential to acknowledge that the journey to healing and empowerment often feels like stepping into the unknown. It is not a well-trodden path, and it can indeed feel lonely at times. This loneliness comes from releasing a lifetime's worth of pain, patterns, and beliefs that have been part of your identity for so long. You are stepping out of the shadows, letting go of what has been familiar, even if it has caused you suffering.

In doing so, you may find yourself disconnected from the person you once were, unsure of who you are becoming, and uncertain of how you should feel. You are shedding layers of yourself that once acted as armor, and without them, the vulnerability can feel overwhelming. The people around you may not fully understand this shift, which can add to the feeling of isolation. But this is where the true transformation happens—when you allow yourself to sit with the discomfort, to navigate those uncharted emotions, and to trust that on the other side of this release is a stronger, more authentic version of yourself.

Often, we underestimate the power of choice in our lives. We may feel trapped by circumstances, limited by our beliefs, or constrained by our past experiences. However, the truth is that we have more choices than we often realize. Every moment presents an opportunity to choose differently, to break free from old patterns, and to step into a new way of being.

Consider the areas of your life where you feel stuck or limited. What symptom or symptoms are you suffering from the most? If you took a moment to separate yourself from that symptom, what new thoughts or feelings can you envision or replace them with? What steps can you take to move towards those possibilities? This journey is about expanding your perspective and recognizing that you are not confined to the path you have been on, regardless of what you have been told or taught. There are countless roads to explore, each offering its own unique opportunities for growth and transformation.

EMBRACING THE UNKNOWN

The road less traveled can be daunting because it requires us to embrace uncharted territory. It challenges us to step out of our comfort zones and trust in the process of life. But it is on this road that we discover our true potential and the depth of our resilience.

As you continue your journey, remember that you are not alone. There is a community of like-minded individuals who also desire to break free from the constraints of victim consciousness, to experience life without PMDD, and to create a life of purpose and fulfillment. Together, we can support and inspire each other to take the road less traveled and embrace the limitless possibilities that await us.

Let this serve as an invitation to explore your choices, to trust in your ability to create change, and to embark on the path that leads to your highest self. You are the medicine. You are your greatest teacher. Everything you need and want is already within you and available to you.

As I stood at the crossroads making these very shifts in my own healing journey, I began to see the luteal phase was not a curse, but it is like a magnifying glass that illuminated my deepest unmet needs and unresolved pains. Month after month, this phase brought to light the shadows within me, asking me to pay attention, listen, and understand the messages my body was sending.

The luteal phase is marked by a heightened sensitivity that can feel overwhelming. For those with PMDD, this sensitivity is amplified, turning what might be minor irritations for others into monumental challenges.

Have you ever taken the time to look at your responses outside of your luteal phase and reflect on your responses? I began to see that there was such an overdramatization coming up and out of me compared to the minor event that had occurred. Have you ever asked yourself that? Why did I respond that way and feel it so deeply?

Think of the luteal phase as a discerning yet firm mentor. During this time, our body and mind become more sensitive to the gaps between our authentic selves and the life we are leading. This phase serves as a spotlight, illuminating the internal pains that you might otherwise overlook.

For me, the luteal phase became a mirror reflecting my inner world with stark clarity. I could not escape the emotional and physical turmoil that arose each month. I began to ask myself: What is my body trying to tell me? What unresolved issues are coming to the surface? These were not easy questions to face. They required me to dig deep into my past, my emotions, and my experiences. I realized that the anger, sadness, and anxiety I felt were not just random emotions I was experiencing again; they were signals from my body, urging me to address the parts of my life that were out of balance.

THE MAGNIFYING GLASS

As my luteal phase approached each month, I started to see patterns. The same issues would resurface, like clockwork. Arguments with loved ones, feelings of inadequacy, and deep-seated fears would come to the forefront. It was as if PMDD was holding up a magnifying glass to these aspects of my life, demanding my attention.

This realization was both daunting and liberating. It made me understand that PMDD was not just a hormone-sensitive disorder; it was a messenger. My body was not betraying me; it was communicating with me in the only way it knew how. The luteal phase was shining a spotlight on the areas of my life that needed attention, healing, and compassion.

YOUR INWARD CALL

This phase, with all its intensity, became a call to inner work. It invited me to explore my emotions deeply, to understand their origins, and to address the unmet needs they revealed. It was a journey into the depths of my soul, where I had to confront my fears, acknowledge my pain, and embrace my vulnerabilities. My luteal phase was asking me to be present with my emotions, to feel them fully, to question their origins, and to use them as a guide for personal growth.

I invite you to look at your luteal phase with new eyes. Instead of seeing it as a time of complete dread, see it as an opportunity for profound self-exploration. Pay attention to the emotions that arise, the thoughts that persist, and the patterns that repeat. These are not just symptoms to manage; they are messages to understand.

Let's take a moment to tune in and listen to the wisdom of your luteal phase. Close your eyes, breathe deeply, and allow yourself to quiet the noise around you. Just maybe it would sound something like this:

Hello beautiful and brave one,

I am your luteal phase, your inner autumn. I come to you with a purpose, not to burden but to reveal. In my presence, I ask you to pause and listen, to reflect on what lies beneath the surface of your day-to-day life.

I ask you: What emotions have you been suppressing? The irritability, the sadness, the anger—they are not random; they are messages. They are calling you to acknowledge what you have avoided, to confront the truths that demand your attention.

What unmet needs are showing up in your body and mind? I amplify your discomfort not to harm you but to make the whispers of your soul impossible to ignore. Are you honoring yourself, your boundaries, your desires? Or are you stretching yourself too thin, saying yes when you mean no, and silencing your inner voice?

I urge you to ask: What parts of your life feel misaligned? The tension and overwhelm you feel may be pointing to relationships, commitments, or patterns that no longer serve you. What can you release to make space for what truly nourishes you?

I am not your enemy—I am your mirror. I reflect on your deepest beliefs and truths and show you where healing and growth are needed. In this sacred season of reflection, I ask you to lean in, embrace the discomfort, and trust that within it lies the wisdom you need to reclaim your balance and your truth.

Simply sit with it, feel it, and notice how this feels for you. There is no need to judge or fix—just listen. What was your experience?

Allow yourself to be curious, explore this time without judgment, and embrace the wisdom that is being offered to you.

This journey is not about finding quick fixes or easy answers. It is about delving deep into your unique inner world, listening to what is coming up, understanding the messages your body is sending, and beginning the process of true healing from within. Trust in the wisdom of your luteal phase, and let it guide you toward a deeper understanding of yourself and your needs.

In this sacred space of self-exploration, you may find the clarity and strength you need to navigate your journey with PMDD. Remember, you are not alone. We are in this together, and together, we will uncover the insights that lie within.

UNVEILING LIFE THEMES

My luteal phase often felt like a cruel, recurring nightmare. Month after month, like clockwork, I would feel the sabotage roll in, taking over my thoughts and actions. It was as if I had become a different person, someone I hardly recognized. The symptoms were not just physical; they were emotional tsunamis that left me feeling like a monster, a horrible mother, and my own worst enemy. But as I began to pay closer attention, I realized that these symptoms were revealing something deeper, something I needed to understand and address, something I neglected for far too long.

I started noticing recurring life themes that surfaced during my luteal phase. The same issues, fears, doubts, and insecurities would bubble up to the surface. It was like my body and mind conspired to bring these issues to my attention, demanding that I face them head-on.

The voice of sabotage was loud and relentless. It would tell me I was not good enough, that I was failing as a mother, that I was destined to be alone and unhappy. These thoughts would invade my mind, overpowering any sense of rationality or self-worth. But I began to see a pattern in these sabotaging thoughts. They were not random; they were deeply rooted in past experiences, unresolved traumas, and suppressed emotions.

For me, this journey of discovery was both painful and enlightening. I had to face my deepest fears and insecurities and confront the parts of myself that I had been avoiding for so long. But in doing so, I began to understand that my luteal phase was not my enemy. It was a mirror, reflecting the parts of myself that needed healing and attention.

I know how isolating and overwhelming it can feel to be trapped in this cycle. I want you to know that you are not alone. Your symptoms are not a sign of failure or inadequacy. You are not broken. You are not cursed. You were not born this way. Everything that you experience during your luteal phase are signals and guides, urging you to look deeper, to understand yourself better, and to awaken you on a sacred journey of healing and self-discovery.

OK, So What Are These Signals?

These signals, which manifest as your symptoms, are intense, turbulent, and multifaceted, affecting both your physical and emotional well-being. They may show up as severe mood swings, feelings of depression or hopelessness, intense anger or irritability, heightened anxiety or tension, and a deep sensitivity to rejection. You might notice a decreased interest in activities you usually enjoy, difficulty concentrating, overwhelming fatigue, or disrupted energy levels. Changes in appetite or sleep patterns, along with physical discomforts like bloating, breast tenderness, headaches, or joint and muscle pain, can further compound the experience. These symptoms can make you feel as though you are out of control as if your mind and body are betraying you. Yet, they are not random or arbitrary—they are intricately linked to your overall well-being and life experiences, urging you to pause, reflect, and listen to what your body is trying to communicate.

WHERE ARE THESE SYMPTOMS COMING FROM?

Our bodies are intricate storytellers, holding onto the imprints of our lived experiences—both seen and unseen. Dr. Bessel van der Kolk's phrase, "the body keeps the score," highlights this remarkable phenomenon, where our bodies serve as silent witnesses to everything we endure. These imprints are not limited to the monumental traumas we often associate with the word; they encompass any experience that leaves a negative emotional or physical mark on us. It could be the sting of rejection, the weight of unmet expectations, or even the chronic stress of daily life.

When these experiences go unprocessed, our bodies store them in subtle ways—through tension in our muscles, digestive issues, chronic pain, or even cyclical conditions like PMDD. Our emotional states, too, become intertwined with these stored memories, manifesting as unexplained anxiety, irritability, or even fatigue.

This connection between mind and body is both complex and profound. While we may not consciously remember every difficult moment, our bodies hold the memory, responding with fight, flight, freeze, or fawn patterns when triggered. These responses can be automatic, making us feel as though we are reliving old wounds, even if we cannot pinpoint the source.

The traditional definition of trauma refers to a deeply distressing or disturbing experience that overwhelms an individual's ability to cope, often causing feelings of helplessness, fear, or a sense of losing control. Trauma can result from events such as accidents, natural disasters, abuse, violence, or significant loss.

Psychologically, trauma is understood as any event that creates emotional or psychological harm and leaves a lasting impact on an individual's mental and emotional well-being. According to the American Psychological Association (APA), trauma is "an emotional response to a terrible event like an accident, rape, or natural disaster" and can manifest in physical, emotional, or behavioral reactions such as shock, denial, or longer-term symptoms like flashbacks and emotional detachment.

Trauma manifests in various forms, each shaped by the nature and duration of the experience. Acute trauma stems from a single, isolated event, often leaving a sharp and immediate emotional or psychological impact. Chronic trauma, on the other hand, arises from prolonged exposure to distressing circumstances, such as enduring abuse or living through war, fostering a persistent state of stress and hypervigilance. Complex trauma involves repeated or prolonged exposure to multiple, varied traumatic experiences, creating deep and layered emotional and psychological wounds. These different forms of trauma profoundly influence an individual's sense of safety, self-worth, and ability to form healthy relationships. If left unaddressed, trauma can lead to debilitating conditions like Post-Traumatic Stress Disorder (PTSD) or anxiety disorders, emphasizing the critical need for understanding and healing.

REDEFINING TRAUMA

A holistic definition of trauma expands on the traditional view by recognizing trauma not only as an event but also as the individual's internal response to that event. It encompasses the physical, emotional, mental, and spiritual impact of the experience. Holistically, trauma is understood as anything that overwhelms a person's capacity to cope, disrupts their sense of safety, and creates long-term disturbances in how they relate to themselves and the world. This view sees trauma as not just a psychological wound but also something stored in the body and reflected in behavior, relationships, and even physical health.

Gabor Maté, a renowned physician and trauma expert, has greatly influenced the holistic understanding of trauma. His definition extends beyond immediate, catastrophic events to include early-life experiences, neglect, and emotional wounds that shape how we view ourselves and the world. Maté suggests that trauma is not necessarily what happens to us but what happens inside us as a result of what happened to us. He focuses on how trauma disconnects individuals from their true selves, impacting emotional and physical health.

According to Maté, trauma can manifest in various forms, such as chronic stress, addiction, depression, and physical illnesses, because the body and mind are intimately connected. He emphasizes that unresolved trauma can disrupt our nervous system and be stored in the body, causing long-term suffering. Healing trauma, in his view, requires reintegration of the mind and body, compassion for oneself, and the re-establishment of safety and connection. In Maté's approach, trauma is not just a psychological or emotional response but a holistic disturbance that affects every facet of our being, requiring a comprehensive approach to healing.

Here are some examples of such subtle yet impactful traumas:

1. **Childhood Emotional Neglect**: Growing up without adequate emotional support, validation, or connection can leave deep emotional scars. When a child's emotional needs are ignored or dismissed, they may internalize feelings of unworthiness and invisibility. This neglect can create a pervasive sense of being unsupported, affecting self-esteem and emotional regulation well into adulthood.

2. **Chronic Stress from Work or Relationships**: Ongoing stress from demanding work environments or strained relationships can wear down our resilience. When stress becomes a constant part of daily life, it triggers a chronic state of heightened alertness and tension. This continuous stress response can lead to physical ailments, anxiety, and a diminished ability to cope with new stressors.

3. **Feeling Unsupported or Misunderstood**: Consistently feeling unsupported or misunderstood by those around us can create a sense of isolation and loneliness. This lack of support can be especially damaging when it occurs in significant relationships, such as with family,

friends, or partners. Over time, this can erode our sense of belonging and security, leading to feelings of alienation and depression.

4. **Repeated Feelings of Rejection or Failure:** Experiencing repeated rejection, or failure can significantly impact our self-worth and motivation. Whether it is in personal relationships, academic pursuits, or career endeavors, repeated setbacks can create a fear of failure and an aversion to taking risks. This can lead to a cycle of avoidance and self-doubt, limiting personal and professional growth.

ACCUMULATION AND MANIFESTATION OF TRAUMA

These experiences can accumulate over time and manifest as symptoms during the luteal phase, as though everything stored within us rises to the surface and spills into every area of our lives. This heightened sensitivity often results in a range of physical and emotional symptoms. Increased irritability may appear, driven by unresolved emotional wounds and unmet needs, making small stressors feel overwhelming and triggering intense emotional reactions. Feelings of anxiety and depression can also intensify as the accumulation of unmet needs and emotional neglect collide with hormonal changes during the luteal phase, amplifying these emotions. Additionally, chronic stress and emotional suppression often manifest physically, leading to headaches, muscle tension, fatigue, and other somatic symptoms. These physical discomforts tend to become more pronounced during the luteal phase, making them harder to ignore and adding to the overall sense of overwhelm.

Unmet needs are the unfulfilled or unsupported aspects of our lives that create a sense of imbalance and dissatisfaction. These can include a lack of emotional connection, feeling unappreciated, or not dedicating enough time to self-care. When these needs go unmet over time, they generate stress and emotional discomfort that often manifest as physical or emotional symptoms. For instance, a lack of emotional connection can lead to feelings of loneliness and isolation, contributing to sadness and emptiness that become more pronounced during the luteal phase. Feeling unappreciated can undermine self-esteem, fostering a sense of worthlessness and emotional pain that may appear as irritability or resentment. Similarly, neglecting self-care results in physical and emotional burnout, where accumulated stress leaves us more vulnerable to anxiety and depression, particularly during the heightened sensitivity of the luteal phase.

Emotional imprints are the lasting effects of past emotional experiences that shape how we respond to situations in the present. These imprints are created through repeated exposure to specific emotions or circumstances, forming subconscious patterns that guide our reactions to similar experiences in the future. They can heighten our sensitivity to triggers, making us more reactive to anything that reminds us of past traumas or unmet needs. This heightened sensitivity often becomes particularly intense during the luteal phase, leading to amplified emotional responses. Emotional imprints also contribute to recurring emotional patterns, such as anxiety, anger, or sadness, which are further intensified by the hormonal fluctuations of the luteal phase.

THE COMPOUNDED WEIGHT

In my observance, PMDD worsens over time because it thrives on the accumulation of unresolved emotions, suppressed experiences, and the compounded weight of life's changes. This perspective aligns not only with my personal history of PMDD but also with the experiences of many of my clients. It often seems that PMDD symptoms escalate to an entirely new level following a significant life change or event. What may initially present as a subtle feeling of being "off" gradually evolves into something overwhelming and unbearable as each passing year adds more layers of stress, unmet needs, and unprocessed emotions. Life transitions—whether it is getting married, moving, going to college, having children, experiencing loss, or watching your children leave for college—act as triggers, amplifying symptoms and making the emotional burden feel heavier.

There may even be years when PMDD feels relatively dormant or easier to manage—a luteal phase that does not feel as intense because of a period of peace or contentment in life. But when life shifts—a new stressor, transition, or emotional challenge—it can reignite our emotional imprints with renewed intensity, reminding us that the unresolved emotional weight remains.

One might even argue that by the time we reach perimenopause, the turbulence of the hormone shifts becomes almost impossible to ignore. All the emotions, experiences, and stresses we have carried for years finally demand acknowledgment, creating a perfect storm of hormonal and emotional upheaval. The body can no longer bear the unspoken weight and suppressed feelings resurface with greater intensity. This underscores the importance of addressing the root causes early on—breaking the cycle of suppression and giving ourselves the space to heal—before the compounded pain becomes too much to bear.

RECURRING LIFE THEMES: WHAT IS YOUR BODY TELLING YOU?

Were all these symptoms inward manifestations of my suppressed inner world? As I started to pay attention to my symptoms, I noticed that certain themes kept resurfacing. These were not just random occurrences; they were patterns highlighting areas of my life that needed attention. The recurring nature of these symptoms made me realize that my body was trying to communicate something important, urging me to look deeper and address the underlying issues.

THE NEED FOR SELF-WORTH

During my luteal phase, I often felt a deep sense of inadequacy and self-doubt. This was not just a fleeting emotion; it was a profound and persistent feeling that would envelop me; it felt like there was a black cavern of void in me. A pitch-black endless pit. My mind would flood with memories of times when I felt like I was not enough—failed attempts, criticisms from others, and my own harsh self-judgments. It was as if my body was replaying these moments to highlight my struggle with self-worth.

I began to see that these feelings were not isolated incidents but part of a broader narrative that I had internalized over the years. The luteal phase amplified these feelings, making it impossible for me to ignore them any longer. It was my body's way of telling me that I needed to work on loving and valuing myself to build a healthier relationship with my self-esteem.

EMOTIONAL NEGLECT

Feelings of being unsupported or misunderstood would peak during my luteal phase. I would find myself craving validation and empathy, feeling like no one understood what I was going through. These emotions would often lead to intense loneliness and frustration.

Reflecting on these feelings, I realized that they were rooted in past experiences where my emotional needs were not met. Perhaps it was the lack of emotional support during my younger years or the times when I felt dismissed or invalidated by those close to me. My luteal phase was bringing these unresolved emotions to the forefront, urging me to address the emotional neglect I had experienced.

By recognizing this pattern, I began to understand. It became a call to nurture my own emotional well-being, practice self-compassion, and validate my own feelings rather than rely solely on external sources.

I know how isolating and overwhelming it can feel to be trapped in this cycle of recurring symptoms. It is worth repeating; I want you to know that these symptoms are not random; they are messages from your body, asking you to pay attention to areas of your life that need attention, healing, and care. By listening to these signals and making these connections, you can begin to address the underlying issues and make powerful and meaningful changes.

During my luteal phase, one recurring theme that always screamed in my head was that I am not enough, meaning I carried a persistent belief that no matter what you do or achieve, you are inherently inadequate or unworthy of love, acceptance, or success. This left a profound imbalance between my work and home life. Fatigue and anxiety about work became constant companions, deeply affecting my overall well-being. This imbalance was not merely about long hours or heavy workloads; it reflected the emotional and mental toll that work was taking on me, spilling over into every aspect of my life.

At work, I was consumed by the anxiety of overperformance. I constantly feared making mistakes or losing my job, leading to a relentless cycle of hyper-vigilance and perfectionism. I would second-guess every decision, striving to prove my worth and avoid failure. This pressure was emotionally draining, leaving me mentally spent by the end of the day.

By the time I arrived home, the weight of exhaustion was unbearable. I was irritable and short-tempered, snapping at my daughters for the smallest things. These moments filled me with guilt, as I knew they deserved my patience and presence, but I felt too depleted to give it. This guilt only added to my emotional burden, creating a vicious cycle of fatigue, frustration, and regret.

The imbalance between work and home life created palpable tension, affecting my relationships and interactions. My daughters could sense my fatigue and frustration, and this strain weighed heavily on my heart. Fatigue was not just physical—it was a deep, soul-crushing exhaustion that drained my joy and made even simple tasks feel insurmountable. This kind of emotional toll left me feeling helpless and hopeless, struggling to see a way out.

Balancing the demands of my career, single motherhood, and my own individual needs felt impossible. I was pulled in so many directions, each role demanding more than I felt capable of giving. This relentless pressure left me feeling inadequate in every area, unable to fully meet the expectations of any role. The imbalance was more than just a logistical challenge; it was an emotional and mental struggle that left me questioning how to find harmony in a life that felt so overwhelming.

Journaling during your luteal phase is a powerful tool for uncovering and releasing underlying thoughts and emotions that may otherwise remain buried. When you take the time to write down your feelings, symptoms, and experiences, you create a safe space to explore what your body and mind are trying to communicate. Patterns and recurring themes often appear, revealing the unspoken needs, fears, or unresolved emotions that lie beneath the surface. This process allows you to identify areas of your life that require attention and fosters a deeper understanding of yourself.

Through journaling, you can begin to release the weight of these emotions by giving them a voice. Writing them down creates clarity, offering a new perspective and often leading to insights that empower you to take action or make meaningful changes. It is not just about cataloging symptoms—it's about connecting with your inner world and allowing your thoughts to flow freely without judgment.

Here are a few questions to guide your journaling practice:

- ✧ What recurring thoughts or emotions arise during your luteal phase?

_____

_____

_____

- ✧ Are there specific triggers or situations that intensify your symptoms or emotional responses?

_____

_____

_____

✧ What is your body asking for at this moment—rest, nourishment, boundaries, or something else?

_____

_____

_____

✧ What unmet needs, emotional imprints, or unresolved experiences might be contributing to how you feel right now?

_____

_____

_____

✧ How do you speak to yourself during this phase, and how might you show yourself more compassion?

_____

_____

_____

Allow yourself to write openly and honestly, knowing that the process itself is healing. Each entry is a step toward understanding and addressing the deeper layers of your experience.

By understanding what your symptoms are revealing, you can start to address the root causes and make positive changes in your life. Remember, you are not alone on this journey. Many are walking this path, learning to listen to our bodies and heal from within. Together, we can transform our pain into a source of strength and wisdom.

Ritualistic Responses: The Hidden Impact of Trauma on Mind and Body

As we continue to explore the symptoms of PMDD, it is crucial to recognize how our repetitive responses have become ritualistic, automatic behaviors that our mind and body initiate without conscious thought. These responses are more than just habits; they are deeply ingrained trauma responses that can have significant negative impacts on our mental and physical health. By looking deeper, we can understand what our bodies are trying to tell us and how these responses have become part of our everyday lives.

UNDERSTANDING TRAUMA RESPONSES

Trauma responses are ways our bodies and minds react to perceived threats based on past experiences. These responses are often categorized into four main types: fight, flight, freeze, and fawn. Each of these responses has distinct characteristics and can manifest in many ways, especially in those of us dealing with PMDD. Let's break down each trauma response, explore what prompts these reactions, and delve into what is happening in our brains and bodies during these moments.

WHAT IS HAPPENING IN THE BRAIN AND NERVOUS SYSTEM?

When we experience trauma responses, our brain and nervous system play a central role. The amygdala, the brain's fear center, detects a threat and signals the hypothalamus to activate the stress response, triggering the release of stress hormones like adrenaline and cortisol. These hormones prepare the body for immediate action—whether to fight, flee, freeze, or fawn—by activating the sympathetic nervous system (SNS). This leads to an increase in heart rate, blood pressure, and respiration, while the parasympathetic nervous system (PNS), responsible for relaxation, is suppressed. This imbalance keeps the body in a heightened state of alertness and stress.

The nervous system, including the central nervous system (CNS) and peripheral nervous system (PNS), functions as the body's command and communication center. The CNS made up of the brain and spinal cord, processes information and coordinates the body's activities, while the PNS connects the CNS to the rest of the body, enabling responses to stimuli. Together, they regulate everything from basic functions like heartbeat and breathing to complex reactions to external stressors, ensuring the body maintains homeostasis and adapts to its environment.

THE FOUR TRAUMA RESPONSES

1. **Fight Response**

The fight response is characterized by a need to confront and challenge the perceived threat. This can manifest as anger, irritability, or even aggression. When we perceive a threat, our body releases stress hormones like adrenaline and cortisol, preparing us to stand our ground.

Example 1: Husbands and Partners During the luteal phase, you might find yourself snapping at your partner over seemingly trivial issues. A misplaced item or an offhand comment can trigger an intense reaction. This is your body's way of trying to regain control in a situation where you feel vulnerable or misunderstood.

Example 2: Children and Home Life The fight response can also appear when dealing with your children. Simple requests or minor misbehaviors can set off a cascade of frustration and anger, leaving you feeling like a monster afterward. Your body is responding to the perceived stress of being overwhelmed and not having enough support.

Example 3: Career At work, you might react strongly to criticism or feel the need to defend your decisions aggressively. This response is your body's way of protecting you from perceived threats to your competence and job security.

2. **Flight Response**

The flight response involves an urge to escape or avoid the perceived threat. This can manifest as anxiety, restlessness, or a constant need to stay busy. Your body is flooded with stress hormones, preparing you to flee from danger.

Example 1: Husbands and Partners You might find yourself withdrawing from your partner, avoiding conversations, or spending more time away from home. This is your body's way of trying to escape the stress and emotional overwhelm.

Example 2: Children and Home Life At home, you might feel the need to constantly clean or organize, using busyness as a way to distract yourself from underlying anxiety. Your body is trying to create a sense of control in an environment where you feel overwhelmed.

Example 3: Career In your career, you might take on extra projects or work longer hours to avoid dealing with stress at home or within yourself. This constant busyness is your body's attempt to flee from emotional discomfort.

3. **Freeze Response**

The freeze response is characterized by a feeling of being stuck or paralyzed. You might find it hard to make decisions or take action, feeling overwhelmed by your emotions and unable to move forward. This response is your body's way of trying to protect you by shutting down.

> **Example 1**: Husbands and Partners In your relationship, you might find yourself shutting down during conflicts, unable to speak or defend yourself. This is your body's way of protecting you from further emotional harm by becoming still and unresponsive.
>
> **Example 2**: Children and Home Life At home, you might feel paralyzed by the demands of parenting, unable to address issues or make decisions. This response leaves you feeling helpless and trapped.
>
> **Example 3**: Career At work, you might procrastinate or avoid important tasks, feeling stuck and unable to move forward. This paralysis is your body's way of protecting you from perceived threats of failure or criticism.

4. **Fawn Response**

The fawn response involves trying to appease or please the perceived threat to avoid conflict. This can manifest as people-pleasing, difficulty saying no, or putting others' needs above your own. Your body is trying to ensure safety by keeping harmony and avoiding confrontation.

> **Example 1:** Husbands and Partners You might go out of your way to meet your partner's needs, even when it is detrimental to your own well-being. This is your body's way of trying to prevent conflict and maintain peace.
>
> **Example 2:** Children and Home Life With your children, you might overcompensate by giving in to their demands or avoiding setting boundaries. This response aims to keep the peace and avoid further stress.
>
> **Example 3**: Career At work, you might take on more tasks than you can handle, constantly seeking approval and validation from your superiors. This is your body's way of ensuring safety by being seen as indispensable.

For those with PMDD, these stress responses can become disproportionately triggered by the hormonal changes that precede menstruation. Instead of a true threat, it is the internal fluctuations of hormones like estrogen and progesterone that can set off these responses, leading to heightened states of anxiety or irritability. This misfiring can make everyday stressors feel insurmountable, turning normal challenges into overwhelming obstacles.

Reflection Questions

As you reflect on these trauma responses, consider the following questions - here are 10 reflective questions to explore and better understand trauma responses:

1. What situations or interactions tend to trigger a strong emotional or physical reaction in me?

   _____

   _____

   _____

2. How does my body feel when I am in a heightened state of stress or alertness? (e.g., tightness, racing heart, shallow breath)

   _____

   _____

   _____

3. Do I notice any recurring patterns in how I respond to stressful situations—fight, flight, freeze, or fawn?

   _____

   _____

   _____

4. What past experiences might be influencing how I react to certain triggers today?

   _____

   _____

   _____

5. In moments of distress, what thoughts or beliefs arise about me or others?

   _____

   _____

   _____

6. How do my trauma responses affect my relationships with those around me?

_____
_____
_____

7. What coping mechanisms (healthy or unhealthy) or behaviors do I rely on when I feel overwhelmed or unsafe?

_____
_____
_____

8. Are there times when my responses have helped me navigate difficult situations, and how do I feel about that?

_____
_____
_____

9. What messages might my body be trying to communicate to me through these responses?

_____
_____
_____

10. How can I create moments of safety and grounding for myself when I feel activated or triggered?

_____
_____
_____

These questions invite self-awareness and insight, helping you better understand your responses and begin to process them with compassion.

By seeing these responses through a different lens, we can begin to understand their origins and impacts on our lives. This awareness is another step towards breaking the cycle and finding healthier ways to cope with the challenges of PMDD. Remember, this journey is about understanding and compassion for yourself as you navigate these complex and deeply rooted responses.

THE NERVOUS SYSTEM AND PMDD

PMDD affects not only physical health but also emotional well-being through its profound interaction with the nervous system, which regulates stress responses and overall balance. In a healthy state, the nervous system maintains homeostasis, fostering calmness and resilience. However, in PMDD, the nervous system often becomes dysregulated, struggling to return to equilibrium after stress, which intensifies symptoms like heightened sensitivity, anxiety, and mood swings.

Hormonal fluctuations during the luteal phase further disrupt this balance. The sharp decline in estrogen and progesterone destabilizes the nervous system and neurotransmitters like serotonin, deepening symptoms of depression, irritability, and stress. This interplay underscores the critical connection between PMDD and nervous system dysregulation.

Recognizing this link opens doors to effective management through holistic approaches. Practices such as mindfulness, meditation, and prayer can help re-establish nervous system balance, providing relief from symptoms and fostering a calmer, more harmonious state of being.

MINDFUL TECHNIQUES

Mindfulness, meditation, breathwork, and prayer serve as powerful practices for emotional and physiological regulation. These timeless techniques offer a way to bring our inner world into harmony with the outer, creating a sense of peace and grounding even amidst the storm of hormonal fluctuations. Through mindfulness, we cultivate awareness of our thoughts, emotions, and body, allowing us to observe without judgment. Meditation deepens this awareness, helping us find stillness in the chaos, while prayer adds a spiritual dimension, inviting divine guidance and support. Together, these practices foster tranquility, balance, and the strength to navigate life's challenges with grace.

MINDFULNESS

Mindfulness is the practice of fully focusing on the present moment with acceptance and without judgment. It involves being aware of your surroundings, thoughts, emotions, and bodily sensations without labeling them as good or bad. Key aspects include present-moment awareness, non-judgmental observation, and acceptance of experiences as they are. Mindfulness can be practiced through simple activities like mindful breathing, eating, or walking, fostering a sense of calm, clarity, and improved emotional regulation.

MEDITATION

Meditation is referenced in the Bible; it emphasizes reflection, focus, and communion with God. The Hebrew word often translated as "meditate" is hagah, which means to murmur, ponder, or reflect deeply. Another word, siach, conveys the idea of contemplation or speaking thoughtfully. Throughout Scripture, meditation is portrayed as a practice of focusing on God's Word, His works, and His character. For instance, Psalm 1:2 describes the blessed individual as one who meditates on God's law day and night, signifying a continuous, intentional engagement with divine truths. God encourages meditation as a way to align our hearts and minds with His will, offering spiritual clarity, strength, and peace.

Meditation, in a broader sense, is a practice of intentional focus and reflection that fosters concentration, clarity, and emotional balance. It offers a way to deepen understanding of one's inner experiences and cultivate a sense of peace and connection. While techniques may vary, the essence of meditation lies in creating space to quiet the mind, observe thoughts and feelings without judgment, and center oneself. This practice nurtures emotional well-being, reduces stress, and enhances inner harmony, aligning well with the spiritual principles of reflection and intentional focus.

Mindfulness and meditation can be practiced formally or informally, offering benefits such as stress reduction, improved emotional regulation, enhanced focus and concentration, and a greater sense of overall well-being. These practices promote relaxation, increase emotional awareness, and cultivate inner peace and balance in daily life.

For those navigating PMDD, mindfulness and meditation serve as powerful tools for finding balance. They help align internal rhythms with the external world, offering calm and stability amidst the hormonal fluctuations of the condition. With consistent practice, these techniques foster a greater sense of resilience and empowerment, significantly improving overall well-being.

BREATHWORK

Breathwork refers to intentional breathing exercises designed to regulate the nervous system, enhance emotional balance, and promote physical and mental well-being. During the luteal phase, when PMDD symptoms like anxiety, irritability, and fatigue can intensify, breathwork serves as a grounding tool to calm the mind, release tension, and restore a sense of inner peace. Techniques such as deep diaphragmatic breathing or rhythmic patterns can reduce stress and support emotional regulation, helping to alleviate the heightened sensitivity of this phase.

Interestingly, breathwork has also been linked to spiritual practices, including the ancient Hebrew understanding of the name of God, Yahweh. Some interpretations suggest that the act of breathing—inhale and exhale—mirrors the sound of Yahweh, symbolizing the divine presence in every breath. This connection reinforces the idea that breath is not only a tool for physical and emotional healing but also a sacred act, inviting us to align with the divine and embrace the restorative power of God's presence in moments of stillness and reflection.

Incorporating breathwork during the luteal phase can be both a practical and spiritual practice, fostering balance and offering a reminder of the sacred nature of life's rhythms.

PRAYER

Prayer is a deeply personal spiritual practice that connects us with the divine, a higher power, or our inner selves. It serves as a means of communication to express gratitude, seek guidance, find peace, or ask for strength and support. Whether spoken or silent, structured or spontaneous, prayer transcends words, offering a sacred space for reflection, surrender, and connection.

Key forms of prayer include gratitude prayers, which cultivate appreciation and shift focus from lack to abundance; petition prayers, where we seek help or intervention; and centering prayers, which foster stillness and a deep sense of presence. Confession and forgiveness prayers help release emotional burdens, while prayers for healing focus on restoring physical, emotional, or spiritual well-being. Surrender prayers invite trust in divine wisdom, and affirmative prayers affirm positive truths and intentions. Together, these practices nurture a profound sense of peace, trust, and alignment with something greater than ourselves.

Prayer, mindfulness, meditation, and breathwork offer deeply personal practices that foster peace, self-awareness, and a connection to the divine. These techniques, rooted in both ancient traditions and modern understanding, provide powerful tools for managing the emotional and physical challenges of PMDD. By incorporating these practices, individuals can cultivate inner serenity and resilience, creating a foundation for navigating life with grace.

Scientific research supports the effectiveness of these approaches, highlighting their ability to reduce stress, improve emotional regulation, and enhance overall well-being. By blending the spiritual and the scientific, these practices offer a holistic path to healing and empowerment, allowing individuals to embrace life with greater balance and confidence.

SOMATIC PRACTICES FOR RELEASE

In addition to mindful approaches, somatic practices offer a holistic approach to healing, particularly for individuals managing the challenges of PMDD. These methods focus on the interconnectedness of the mind and body, helping to release stored trauma and promote emotional regulation. Somatic Experiencing (SE) emphasizes body awareness to renegotiate trauma and restore self-regulation, using techniques like grounding exercises, mindful walking, reiki, progressive muscle relaxation, and haptic touch to reduce stress and enhance presence. Movement therapies, such as Kundalini yoga, dance therapy, and traditional yoga, further support healing by encouraging the release of stored emotional and physical tension. By integrating these practices into daily life, individuals can improve their ability to manage stress, foster emotional resilience, and reconnect with their physical selves, creating a pathway toward greater well-being and freedom from trauma.

Take a moment to reflect on the new mindful approaches you might consider exploring. There is a wealth of practices beyond traditional methods, each offering unique ways to support your inward journey. This chapter provides just a glimpse of the possibilities available to help you create a personalized practice, empowering you to transform your relationship with PMDD and embrace a path of healing and self-discovery.

As we wrap up this chapter, remember that the road less traveled is often the one that leads to profound transformation. Embracing new concepts like holistic approaches, insights into trauma, and understanding trauma responses may feel unfamiliar, even daunting, at times. Yet, it is in these uncharted paths that true healing exists. PMDD, with all its complexities, is not just a diagnosis—it is an invitation to pause, reflect, and rediscover the truth of who you are beneath the symptoms. By stepping onto this less-traveled road, you honor not only your struggle but also your strength and resilience. Trust the journey, knowing that every pause, every reflection, and every brave step forward is leading you closer to the life you were always meant to live—whole, free, and deeply connected to yourself.

Chapter Six

YOUR SENSITIVITY IS A GIFT

> *"We can only fully tap into all that our emotional intelligence has to offer when we are able to really sit with what we are feeling, even when what we are feeling is pain. There is a certain kind of magic that comes through pain, for it is where we learn of our power to keep going no matter what we go through."*
> – Cleo Wade

Your sensitivity is not a flaw: it is your profound gift. It is part of you that allows you to feel deeply, connect authentically, and experience the world in vivid and meaningful ways. But for those with PMDD, this sensitivity can feel like a curse, turning into an overwhelming flood of emotions and symptoms that seem to take over your life. It is important to remember that PMDD is not a hormonal imbalance disorder—it is a hormone sensitivity disorder. Your body is not broken; it is responding in a heightened way to hormonal shifts, and that response holds deeper meaning. What if we paused to explore the why behind this sensitivity?

What if your body, through this sensitivity, is trying to reveal something profound about your needs, your emotions, or even the unresolved layers of your past? By asking these questions, we begin to move beyond the symptoms and into a deeper understanding of your body, your mind, and the unique ways they are calling you toward healing and wholeness.

As a child, your sensitivity was your superpower. It shaped the way you saw the world- through vivid colors, deep emotions, and a profound connection to the people and experiences around you. It allowed you to notice the smallest details, feel emotions deeply, and connect in ways others could only dream of. This sensitivity was not a flaw; it was a gift, something uniquely yours that set you apart and made you beautifully authentic. It gave you a richness of experience, a creative spirit, and an ability to empathize and care for others on a profound level.

But somewhere along your timeline, that gift became heavy. Life's challenges, unmet needs, or unresolved pain began to pile on, and what once made you unique started to feel like a curse. Depression, anxiety, and rage have seized this sensitivity and inverted it, twisting it into something unrecognizable. The deep feelings that once connected you to joy and wonder began to overwhelm you with sadness, fear, and anger. Instead of enhancing your life, your sensitivity became a source of pain, creating a cycle of emotional extremes that left you exhausted and disconnected.

PMDD is a thief. The vibrant, intuitive, and creative person you once were starts to fade into the background, replaced by a version of yourself that feels unrecognizable—someone trapped in a pattern of emotional chaos that you could not control. The world, which once felt full of possibility, now feels like a place of dread and unpredictability. It is as if PMDD hijacked your authentic self, leaving you questioning who you are and often your sanity, too.

But here is the truth: that authentic, sensitive, and unique person is still within you. PMDD may distort your experience, but it cannot erase who you truly are. The sensitivity that feels like a burden now is still the same gift that made you special as a child—it simply needs to be nurtured, healed, and reconnected to its purpose. Your deep feelings are not your enemy; they are a guide, a reminder of your ability to feel deeply and live authentically. While PMDD tries to mask this truth, the journey of healing is about unmasking it—rediscovering the power of your sensitivity and using it to reclaim the vibrant, unique person you were always meant to be.

Perhaps you heard things like, "Stop being so dramatic; it's not a big deal," or "Why do you cry over everything? Toughen up!" These words can cut deep, making you feel invalidated. Maybe someone told you,

"You need to learn to take a joke," or "Don't be so sensitive; it's just constructive criticism," further pushing you to question your reactions and feelings. It is possible you were labeled as always overreacting and heard, "Why can't you be more like your sibling?" Such comparisons can leave lasting scars, making you believe that your natural responses were wrong. You might have been told, "You need to grow a thicker skin," or "You worry too much about what others think," adding to your sense of isolation. The comments "You're too emotional; calm down" and "Why do you take everything so personally?" likely made you feel ashamed of your sensitivity, driving you to hide your true self. These experiences from your childhood can shape how you perceive your emotions and responses today, influencing your journey through life and how you manage your mental and emotional health.

As a child, your heightened awareness and deep emotional capacity were not flaws but rather indicators of your empathetic nature. Your ability to feel deeply means you can connect with others on a profound level, offering compassion and understanding that many might not possess. Those tears and emotions were signs of a caring and loving heart, one that is attuned to the subtleties of the world around you. Your sensitivity is the foundation of your kindness, allowing you to notice and respond to the needs of others in ways that are truly meaningful. This gift, when not seen or nurtured properly, can make you feel like the weirdo of your family, the black sheep, the lone wolf, the one who will always be misunderstood, the one that no one will get.

Your creativity, too, is intertwined with your sensitivity. The very emotions that others might have dismissed as overreactions are the same ones that fuel your imagination and artistic expression. Your unique perspective allows you to see beauty and possibility where others might see only the mundane. Being sensitive means you experience the world vividly, and this vividness can translate into a powerful creativity that enriches both your life and the lives of those around you.

Recognizing these aspects of yourself can help you begin to embrace your sensitivity as a strength. It is what makes you uniquely you—empathetic, intuitive, caring, loving, kind, creative, and unique. These qualities are not just positive; they are essential to the fabric of your identity. They are the gifts that enable you to make a profound impact on the world, transforming your sensitivity from a perceived weakness into a celebrated strength.

But what happens when those feelings of being misunderstood and overwhelmed drive you away, when this becomes a life theme where you feel like you don't fit in, you are alone, and no one gets you, when you are constantly told that you are dramatic and too much?

These experiences can have profound impacts on the mind, body, and brain. In the mind, these repeated messages can create deep-seated beliefs about your worth and place in the world. You might start to internalize the idea that you are inherently flawed or that your emotions are a burden to others. This can lead to a pervasive sense of inadequacy and a fear of expressing your true self. Over time, this self-doubt can erode your self-esteem and make you hesitant to engage fully with others, leading to isolation and loneliness.

In the brain, the impact can be equally significant. Persistent feelings of isolation and misunderstanding can alter the brain's structure and function. The limbic system, which is responsible for processing emotions, can become overactive, making it harder to regulate your emotional responses. The prefrontal cortex, which helps with decision-making and social interactions, might become less effective, leading to difficulties in navigating social situations and making choices that align with your well-being.

More importantly, the brain's neural pathways are shaped by repeated experiences and thoughts. If you continually feel like an outsider, your brain can reinforce these pathways, making it more challenging to break out of these patterns. This can create a cycle where the more you feel misunderstood, the more your brain expects and anticipates these experiences, perpetuating feelings of alienation and disconnection.

For many with PMDD, the gift of sensitivity often goes hand in hand with an extraordinary capacity for empathy. This empathy allows you to intuitively sense the emotions of others, feel their pain as if it were your own, and connect with a depth that others may not fully understand. It is as though your sensitivity acts as an antenna, picking up on the unspoken energies and needs around you. While this gift is beautiful, it can also become overwhelming when PMDD heightens your emotional responses, leaving you absorbing not only your struggles but the struggles of those around you. Empathy, when coupled with heightened sensitivity, can feel like a double-edged sword—on one side, it fosters meaningful relationships and profound compassion, but on the other, it can drain your emotional reserves. This correlation between empathy and sensitivity is a powerful reminder that your deep emotional capacity is not a weakness;

it is a strength that, when understood and nurtured, can be one of your greatest assets on the journey toward healing and self-discovery.

Exploring your personal sensitivity and personality can be a transformative step in understanding yourself more deeply and reclaiming your sense of identity, especially if you have been navigating the challenges of PMDD. Sensitivity often shapes how you process the world around you—your emotions, reactions, and even your relationships. By identifying your unique traits, you can gain insight into your strengths, areas of vulnerability, and how to best support yourself. This self-awareness can empower you to work with, rather than against, your nature, making space for healing and growth.

Here are some ways you can start finding your type:

1. **Personality Assessments:** Tools like the Myers-Briggs Type Indicator (MBTI) or the Enneagram can provide valuable insights into your personality and how sensitivity shows up in your life.
2. **Sensory Sensitivity Exploration:** Reflect on how you respond to sensory input. Are you easily overwhelmed by sounds, lights, or textures? This could indicate high sensory sensitivity, which is common among highly sensitive people (HSPs).
3. **Emotional Reflection**: Pay attention to how you process emotions. Do you tend to feel others' emotions deeply? Journaling about your reactions to situations can help identify patterns.
4. **Energy Awareness:** Notice how your energy levels fluctuate around different people or environments. Are you energized by quiet and calm or drained by busy, chaotic settings?
5. **Childhood Clues:** Reflect on your childhood. Were you described as "too emotional", "too much", or "too sensitive"? These early traits often hold keys to understanding your natural tendencies.
6. **Creative Outlets**: Consider how you express yourself creatively. Sensitive personalities often find connection and clarity in art, dance, music, or writing.

Understanding your sensitivity is not about labeling yourself but about recognizing and embracing the unique ways you interact with the world. This awareness can be a powerful tool to help you approach your next luteal phase a bit differently, with more personal awareness, to align with your needs and celebrate the beautiful individuality that makes you who you are.

Understanding your personal sensitivity and personality is deeply connected to the gifts of empathy. Empathy is the ability to feel and understand the emotions of others, to step into their experience, and to sense their joys, struggles, and pain. For an empath—someone with an extraordinary level of this ability—empathy becomes more than a skill; it is a way of being. Empaths not only sense emotions but often absorb them, experiencing the world in profound and intuitive ways. Their connection to people, animals, and nature runs deep as they instinctively tune into the energy around them. This can create a unique bond with the world, fostering compassion, nurturing relationships, and a deep respect for life's interconnectedness.

An empath relates to the world with a heightened sense of awareness. They may feel the sadness in someone's voice before it is expressed, understand the unspoken needs of animals, or find themselves deeply moved by the beauty and rhythms of nature. These gifts often manifest as a calling to care for others, to create harmony, or to bring healing into the world. However, these gifts can also become overwhelming when the empath is unable to fully express themselves or process the emotions they absorb. Suppressed emotions can accumulate, leading to exhaustion, anxiety, or even physical symptoms as the body bears the weight of unprocessed energy.

When empaths do not have the tools to release this emotional burden, their gifts can start to work against them. Instead of being a source of connection and insight, their sensitivity may feel like a curse, leaving them overstimulated, drained, or disconnected from their own needs. They may struggle with boundary-setting, taking on the pain of others as their own, which can lead to resentment, burnout, or a loss of identity. Over time, the gifts of empathy—compassion, intuition, and a deep understanding of others—can be lost to self-protection as the empath withdraws to avoid being overwhelmed.

For an empath to thrive, it is essential to process emotions and pain regularly, allowing the flow of energy to move through them rather than settle within. By understanding their sensitivity, setting boundaries, and honoring their own needs, empaths can reclaim their gifts as a source of strength. When supported, their empathy becomes a powerful force for good, enriching their lives and the lives of those they touch. It is a delicate balance, but one that, when achieved, allows the empath to express their unique gifts fully and live in harmony with themselves and the world around them.

HONORING YOUR SENSITIVITY

In a world that often equates strength with outward success over inner fulfillment, sensitivity can feel like a liability. Yet, it is precisely this sensitivity that is one of our greatest gifts, deserving not of shame but of honor. Learning to embrace and celebrate our sensitive nature is essential for our well-being and personal growth. Honoring your sensitivity begins with self-acceptance.

Recognize that being sensitive is not a flaw or a weakness; it is an integral part of who you are. Sensitivity allows you to experience life more vividly and connect more deeply with others. It is your God-given gift. Accepting this aspect of yourself is the first step toward living authentically and fully. Instead of shaming yourself for feeling things intensely or needing more time to process emotions, give yourself permission to experience your feelings without judgment. Sensitivity often means experiencing a wide range of emotions, from profound joy to deep sorrow. Each of these emotions serves a purpose, offering insights into your inner world and helping you navigate your life with greater awareness and intention.

With PMDD, honoring your sensitivity means recognizing the messages your body and mind are sending you. The emotional intensification during this time is not something to be suppressed or ignored but to be understood and embraced. By noticing and listening to your emotions and feelings, you can address these underlying issues, paving the way for healing and growth. Engage in practices that nurture your sensitive nature. Mindfulness, prayer, meditation, and creative expression can be powerful tools for connecting with your inner self and processing emotions. Again, journaling can help you articulate your thoughts and feelings, providing clarity and a sense of release. These practices allow you to honor your sensitivity by giving it space to exist and be expressed.

Surround yourself with people who understand and appreciate your sensitive nature. Seek out relationships that are supportive and affirming. Being with others who recognize and value your sensitivity can help reinforce the belief that this trait is something to be cherished. Community and connection are vital, and finding a tribe that honors your sensitivity can make a profound difference in how you perceive and embrace this aspect of yourself.

Lastly, celebrate your sensitivity and acknowledge the unique strengths it brings to your life. Your ability to connect deeply with others, perceive the world with rich detail, and navigate life with a profound sense of empathy and compassion are all gifts. Celebrate these qualities and recognize how they contribute positively to your life and the lives of those around you. In honoring your sensitivity, you transform it from a source of shame to a source of strength. You begin to see it not as a burden but as a blessing, a vital part of your identity that enriches your experience of life. By embracing your sensitivity, you open the door to living a more authentic, fulfilled, and connected life.

As we navigate the intricate world between sensitivity and PMDD, we are gifted with a unique perspective. We see the world in deeper colors, feel emotions more intensely, and experience life with a richness that is unique to our nature. While this can undoubtedly make the journey through PMDD more challenging, it also enriches our lives in ways that others might never experience. In the end, our sensitivity, when embraced and understood, can transform from a source of pain into a wellspring of strength. It can lead us to deeper self-knowledge, more meaningful relationships, and a more compassionate approach to life.

With an open heart and mind, you can begin to awaken to the underlying emotions and gifts within you. Embrace your sensitivity as a pathway to self-awareness and personal growth. Honor your feelings, set healthy boundaries, and create supportive environments that nurture your sensitive nature.

Recognize the unique strengths that come with being highly sensitive and use them to enrich your life and the lives of those around you. By viewing the internal turmoil of PMDD as a call back to your original truth and self, you can transform your sensitivity into a source of strength and healing. Reflect on your deepest values and desires and take steps to align your life with your authentic self. Seek out understanding relationships and professional support when needed and remember to practice self-compassion and gratitude. Your sensitivity is a precious gift, and by honoring it, you reclaim the parts of yourself that PMDD has tried to steal. Embrace this journey with courage and openness, and let your sensitivity guide you toward a life of deeper connection, authenticity, and fulfillment.

We are the dancers, the singers, the songwriters, the musicians. We are the painters, the actresses, the filmmakers, the designers. We are the artists who feel life in its fullest expression. We are the intuitive, the empaths, the intercessors, the healers, the nature lovers, the nurturers. We are the nurses, the caretakers, the light workers, those who feel the world with an intensity that others may not understand. But this is what makes us who we are.

Our sensitivity is our gift—it is our unique way of experiencing life. It allows us to see beauty where others might not, to sense what is beneath the surface, to carry the weight of the world, and to transform it into something meaningful. In every role we take on, whether creating, nurturing, or healing, we feel it all. And that is what makes us different, what makes us special. Your sensitivity is not a burden—it is your superpower. It is what allows you to connect, to create, to heal, and to inspire. It is what makes you, you.

This is you. This is me. This is us. We are the beautiful, sensitive souls on this earth. We move through the world with heightened awareness, tuned into energies and emotions that others might pass by. Our hearts beat with the rhythm of creation, and our souls are stirred by the beauty, the pain, the joy, and the complexity of life. We express what cannot be spoken. We are the ones who transform emotion into art, into healing, into something that resonates with others.

It is our sensitivity that empowers us to create, feel, and connect, reminding the world of the depth of the human experience. We are the dreamers and the visionaries, and through us, life becomes art, and art becomes life. And this is why we must heal, because you are a work of art, and the world needs your gift and your light.

Take a moment to pause and reflect on your journey. Allow these questions to guide you deeper into understanding your unique sensitivity and its role in your life:

How have you experienced your sensitivity as both a gift and a burden?

_____

_____

_____

Can you think of moments where it connected you to others or made you feel isolated?

_____

_____

_____

In what ways do you feel PMDD has shaped or distorted your sense of self? Are there parts of you that feel misplaced, hidden, or lost?

_____

_____

_____

Have you ever identified with being the lone wolf or the black sheep in your family or community?

_____

_____

_____

How has that shaped your relationships with others and with yourself? Do you sometimes feel rejected or misunderstood because of your sensitivity?

_____

_____

_____

How does that affect your ability to show up authentically? What emotions surface when you think about reclaiming your true self?

_____

_____

_____

Is there fear, hope, or something else entirely? If you were to fully embrace your sensitivity as a gift, how might your life look different?

_____

_____

Take a few moments to sit with these questions. Write down whatever comes to mind without judgment. Remember, this process is not about fixing yourself—it is about rediscovering and honoring who you truly are.

Chapter SEVEN

DECODING SENSITIVITY, UNDERSTANDING TRIGGERS

> *"As a person thinks, feels, and believes, so is the condition of his or her mind, body, and circumstances."*
> **- Joseph Murphy**

Sensitivity is often seen as a weakness, but from a PMDD perspective, it holds profound wisdom. Sensitivity is like our body's finely tuned radar, alerting us to emotional, physical, or environmental imbalances. When paired with PMDD, this heightened sensitivity often manifests as intense reactions to seemingly small events—what we call triggers. These triggers are not random; they act as mirrors, reflecting unmet needs, unresolved pain, or suppressed emotions within us. Decoding sensitivity means understanding these triggers as invitations to explore what our mind, body, and soul are trying to communicate. By embracing sensitivity, we can begin to untangle the root causes of PMDD symptoms and reclaim the strength hidden in our sensitivity.

When we talk about "triggers," we are referring to a catalyst that elicits a strong emotional or physical response. Being "triggered" means experiencing an intense reaction, often suddenly, due to a specific trigger. These triggers can be external, like a situation or event, or internal, like a thought or memory. When triggered, the body's fight or flight response is activated, releasing stress hormones like cortisol and adrenaline, which prepare the body to respond to perceived threats. This physiological response can be accompanied by emotions like anger, fear, or sadness.

THE NATURE OF TRIGGERS

Triggers are deeply personal signals, unique to each individual, that provoke a strong emotional or physical response. They often arise when current situations resonate with past experiences, tapping into unresolved emotions or memories stored in our subconscious. Like alarm bells, triggers can alert us to areas within ourselves that need attention or healing. In the face of triggers, our immediate reactions might include anger, anxiety, or sadness, revealing the intensity and depth of the underlying issues. Recognizing and understanding these triggers allows us to pause, reflect, and choose a more considered response, ultimately fostering personal growth and emotional resilience.

CONNECTING TRIGGERS TO PMDD SYMPTOMS

For instance, reflect on a recent situation where a seemingly innocent comment from a partner triggers an intense emotional reaction. This reaction might not be proportional to the comment itself, but rather, it is a response to a deeper, unresolved issue that the comment has inadvertently touched upon. The mind recalls past experiences where similar comments might have led to feelings of rejection or unworthiness. The body, in turn, reacts with symptoms such as irritability, anger, or profound sadness, signaling that there is an old wound that needs our attention and healing.

Example 1: Dinner Disagreement

> Imagine you are having dinner with your partner, and they casually mention, "Are you sure you want to eat that much dessert?" This comment, though innocent in intent, instantly triggers a surge of anger and hurt. The intensity of your reaction surprises both of you. You feel a sudden, overwhelming need to defend yourself, and your mind races with thoughts like, "They think I'm fat," or "They don't

love me for who I am." Your body responds with a tightening in your chest, rapid breathing, and an urge to leave the table. This reaction is not just about the dessert; it is tied to past experiences where you felt judged or unworthy, perhaps from childhood or previous relationships where your self-esteem was constantly under scrutiny. The comment has touched a raw nerve, bringing to the surface old wounds that have not yet healed.

Example 2: Career Critique

Consider another scenario where you and your partner are discussing career plans. Your partner suggests, "Maybe you should consider a more stable job, you know, something less risky." This comment, though meant to be practical and caring, sparks an extreme emotional response in you. Suddenly, you feel a wave of anger and panic. You might think, "They don't believe in me," or "I'm not good enough to succeed." Memories flood back of times when you were told you were not capable or when your dreams were dismissed by others. Your body reacts with a tight throat, trembling hands, and a feeling of nausea. This response is far more intense than the comment warrants and highlights a deeper issue of feeling unsupported and undervalued in your ambitions, an old scar that still aches.

ANALYSIS AND REFLECTION

In both scenarios, the comments made by the partner were not intended to hurt. However, they unknowingly struck a chord with deeper, unresolved emotional issues. These intense reactions are signals from our body and mind that there are underlying wounds needing attention. It is crucial to recognize these responses not as overreactions but as indicators of areas within us that require healing and compassion.

Reflection Questions:

1. When have you felt a disproportionate emotional reaction to an innocent comment from someone close to you?

_____

_____

_____

2. Can you identify the deeper unresolved issue that might be triggering such intense responses?

_____

_____

_____

3. What past experiences might be influencing your reaction to these comments?

_____

_____

_____

4. How does your body signal to you that there is an emotional wound needing attention?

_____

_____

_____

5. What steps can you take to begin addressing and healing these underlying issues?

_____

_____

_____

Understanding these reactions through this lens allows for self-compassion and opens the path toward healing and deeper self-awareness.

WHAT IS OUR MIND AND BODY REVEALING?

By understanding the nature of triggers and their connection to PMDD symptoms, we can begin to see that our mind and body are revealing areas where we need to focus our healing efforts. Each symptom is a signpost pointing us toward unresolved emotions, unmet needs, or emotional imprints that are seeking resolution. Rather than viewing our symptoms as purely negative or as something to be eradicated, we can start to see them as opportunities for deeper self-awareness and healing.

THE LUTEAL PHASE - ECHOES OF LITTLE YOU

The luteal phase is a profound revealer of your inner world—a mirror reflecting the deeply rooted beliefs, emotions, and experiences stored within your subconscious mind. Shaped during your earliest years, the subconscious holds the echoes of your younger self, where the little you still resides. These early moments, rich with emotions and impressions, shaped your sense of self and the way you see the world today.

As emotions rise during the luteal phase, they often carry the intensity of past experiences that remain unresolved. These emotions are not arbitrary; they are messengers from your subconscious, inviting you to reconnect with the little you who still holds the pain, joy, or unmet needs of the past. This phase is a sacred opportunity to pause, listen, and begin to heal.

Taking another moment to reflect:

- ✧ What emotions are surfacing for you right now, and what might they be asking of you?
- ✧ Can you notice a pattern or a recurring feeling that has followed you through life?
- ✧ What unmet need or moment from your past might these emotions be pointing toward?
- ✧ If you could sit with the little you inside, what would they say? What do they need from you now to feel safe, loved, and whole?

The luteal phase invites you to gently explore these questions, illuminating the places where your younger self still seeks validation, love, and reassurance. By embracing this phase as a time of connection and healing, you can transform the old narratives that no longer serve you. Let this be a time of compassion and curiosity, where each wave of emotion becomes a guide, helping you release old wounds and step into a renewed sense of clarity, strength, and self-love.

THE FORMATION AND POWER OF THE SUBCONSCIOUS MIND

The subconscious mind is a vast and powerful part of our consciousness, operating beneath the surface of our everyday awareness. It forms over time through our experiences, beliefs, and emotional responses, starting in early childhood and continuing throughout our lives. Unlike the conscious mind, which handles logical thinking and decision-making, the subconscious mind is responsible for automatic behaviors, emotional reactions, and deeply held beliefs that shape our perception of the world.

The formation of the subconscious mind begins with the absorption of information, often in ways we are not fully aware of. This part of the mind forms early in life, primarily during the first seven years when we are highly impressionable and learn primarily through observation and imitation. During this formative period, our brains run primarily in lower brainwave states (such as theta and alpha), which are compared to the states of hypnosis and meditation. This makes young children highly receptive to the beliefs, behaviors, and emotional reactions they observe in their parents and significant others.

As children, we are especially impressionable, and our subconscious absorbs everything—from the words and behaviors of those around us to the emotional tone of our environment. Over time, these experiences create neural pathways in the brain, establishing patterns of thought and behavior that become habitual. These ingrained beliefs and responses are often unexamined, yet they guide our actions and influence our emotions in powerful ways.

By the time a child reaches the age of seven, the subconscious mind is largely formed. Although it continues to develop and adapt throughout our lives, the core programming—the beliefs and patterns established in those early years—remains deeply ingrained. This subconscious programming forms the lens through which we view and interact with the world, shaping our perceptions and reactions in profound ways.

The power of the subconscious mind lies in its ability to influence almost every aspect of our lives without us even realizing it. It is estimated that the subconscious mind governs about 95% of our lives. It controls our habits, emotional responses, and even physical processes like breathing and heart rate. It is also where memories are stored, including suppressed or forgotten experiences that continue to shape our present-day emotions and reactions. The subconscious often speaks to us through dreams, instincts, and gut feelings, offering insights into deeper truths that our conscious mind may overlook. This force holds immense power, shaping our lives in profound and often unnoticed ways. Wild right?

THE POWER OF THE SUBCONSCIOUS MIND

The subconscious mind wields incredible power through its ability to store and retrieve information efficiently, shaping much of our daily behavior without our conscious awareness. It acts as a vast repository for all our memories, habits, and learned behaviors, allowing us to perform routine and complex tasks automatically. This function can be both a gift and a limitation, depending on the type of programming stored within the subconscious.

When positive beliefs are ingrained in the subconscious, they create supportive habits and automatic behaviors that align with our goals and well-being. For instance, someone who subconsciously believes they are capable and deserving of success will naturally seek out opportunities and persevere through challenges with minimal conscious effort. Their internalized belief propels them forward, often without them needing to consciously direct their actions.

On the other hand, negative programming can instill limiting beliefs and self-sabotaging behaviors. For example, if a person has internalized the belief that they are unworthy or incapable, this will manifest in their decisions and actions, often holding them back from reaching their true potential. These deep-seated beliefs can create behavior patterns that reinforce the original programming, trapping the individual in a cycle of self-doubt and underachievement.

THE SUBCONSCIOUS MIND'S PROTECTIVE ROLE

At its core, the subconscious mind's primary function is to protect and ensure our survival. It does this by forming patterns and responses based on early life experiences, interpreting these as essential for our well-being. Most of this programming takes place during childhood, a critical time when the subconscious is particularly open and receptive. During these formative years, the mind and body work in unison to develop survival mechanisms, which then shape our thoughts, feelings, and behaviors throughout life.

These patterns, once established, can serve us in times of need, helping us navigate the world based on past experiences. However, over time, some of these protective mechanisms may become outdated or no longer serve our higher purpose, and they must be reprogrammed for growth, healing, and greater alignment with our true potential.

EARLY CHILDHOOD: THE ABSORBENT MIND

From birth to around seven years old, a child's brain operates predominantly in the theta brainwave state, similar to a state of hypnosis. In this state, the child's mind is incredibly open and impressionable, absorbing vast amounts of information from their environment. This period is known as the "absorbent mind" phase, a term coined by Dr. Maria Montessori. During these years, the subconscious mind records everything—the sights, sounds, emotions, and experiences—creating the foundational programs that will guide future behaviors.

FORMATION OF PATTERNS AND RESPONSES

As children navigate their early years, their subconscious mind is constantly interpreting and storing information. This process involves a few critical steps:

1. **Observation and Absorption:** Children see the actions, reactions, and behaviors of their caregivers and others around them. They absorb the emotional tones, attitudes, and responses they witness.
2. **Interpretation and Meaning-Making**: The subconscious mind interprets these observations and assigns meanings to them. For instance, if a child often receives comfort when crying, the subconscious mind learns that expressing distress leads to receiving care and safety.
3. **Pattern Formation:** Based on these interpretations, the subconscious mind forms patterns and responses. These patterns are automated scripts that the mind will use to navigate future situations. For example, a child who learns that being quiet and compliant avoids conflict will develop a pattern of people-pleasing behavior.

BIOLOGICAL AND PSYCHOLOGICAL MECHANISMS

The formation of these patterns is supported by both biological and psychological mechanisms:

1. Neuroplasticity: During early childhood, the brain is highly plastic or flexible, meaning it can easily form new neural connections. This neuroplasticity allows the subconscious mind to rapidly learn and solidify new patterns based on experiences.
2. Emotional Memory: The amygdala, a part of the brain responsible for processing emotions, plays a significant role in storing emotional memories—strong emotional experiences, whether positive or negative, are imprinted more deeply into the subconscious.
3. Hormonal Influences: Stress hormones such as cortisol and adrenaline are released during intense emotional experiences. These hormones enhance the encoding of these experiences into memory, making the associated patterns more robust.

PROTECTIVE BEHAVIORS AND RESPONSES

The subconscious mind's protective mechanisms are designed to ensure safety and survival by:

1. **Avoidance**: If a child experiences rejection or criticism, the subconscious mind might develop avoidance behaviors to prevent future hurt. For instance, avoiding speaking up in class to avoid potential embarrassment.
2. **Compliance**: To avoid conflict or punishment, a child might learn to comply with authority figures, leading to patterns of people-pleasing and difficulty asserting personal boundaries.
3. **Aggression**: In some cases, the subconscious mind might develop aggressive responses as a defense mechanism against perceived threats learned from observing similar behaviors in the environment.
4. **Withdrawal**: A child who faces overwhelming stress might develop withdrawal behaviors, retreating from social interactions to protect themselves from potential harm.

LONG-TERM IMPACT

While these protective patterns serve an essential function during childhood, ensuring safety and emotional security, they can become self-defeating in adulthood. The subconscious mind, operating with the same patterns formed in early childhood, may continue to trigger these protective responses even when they are no longer appropriate or necessary. For example:

- **Social Anxiety**: A person who learned to avoid judgment by staying quiet might struggle with social anxiety in adulthood, fearing rejection in social settings.
- **Perfectionism**: Someone who received validation through achievement may develop perfectionistic tendencies, constantly striving for success to feel worthy.
- **Relationship Challenges**: Protective behaviors like compliance or aggression can make it difficult to form healthy, balanced relationships.

Understanding the four trauma responses—fight, flight, freeze, and fawn—is crucial, as discussed in the earlier chapter. These responses are deeply ingrained survival mechanisms developed during early experiences to protect us from perceived threats. Recognizing these patterns in our behavior can provide valuable insights into how past traumas continue to influence our present actions and reactions. For instance, the fight response might manifest as aggression or defensiveness, while the flight response can appear as avoidance or anxiety. The freeze response often leads to feelings of helplessness or dissociation, and the fawn response can result in people-pleasing or difficulty setting boundaries. By identifying and understanding these responses, we can begin to address the root causes of our emotional and behavioral patterns, paving the way for healing and growth.

INTEGRATION AND MOVING FORWARD: EMBRACING HEALING AND GROWTH

Discovering and understanding the subconscious mind, our behaviors, and the triggers that activate them is more than an exercise in self-awareness—it is a crucial step toward profound emotional healing and resilience. By delving into the intricacies of our subconscious, we uncover the hidden forces that shape our actions, thoughts, and feelings. This newfound understanding empowers us to recognize the protective patterns formed in our early years, allowing us to address the root causes of our emotional and behavioral responses.

As we learn how the mind works, we can begin to forge a stronger connection between our mind and body. This connection is vital for holistic healing, as it enables us to become more attuned to the signals our body sends us. By paying attention to these signals, we can notice when we are reacting from a place of unresolved trauma or unmet needs and take steps to address and heal these underlying issues.

This journey requires patience, compassion, and a willingness to confront and release the past. However, the rewards are immense—a deeper understanding of ourselves, greater emotional freedom, and the ability to live a more authentic and fulfilling life. As we move forward, let us commit to this path of self-discovery and transformation, knowing that each step brings us closer to the healing and resilience we seek.

As we close this chapter on decoding triggers, we begin to see PMDD through a transformative lens—not as some mystery to endure but as a profound compilation of unhealed traumas, both possibly big but definitely small, held within the subconscious mind. Because, let's face it, we have all experienced trauma on some level. These traumas, carried like an anchoring unseen weight, subtly shape our emotions, reactions, and sense of self. Each trigger becomes a doorway to understanding how these experiences have woven themselves into the fabric of our being, often manifesting as the cyclical storm of PMDD. By acknowledging this connection, we are invited to release judgment of our sensitivity and instead embrace it as a guide toward healing. With every trigger we decode, we step closer to unraveling the layers of hurt, reclaiming ourselves, and rewriting the narrative that PMDD has written in our lives

Chapter EIGHT

THE DEEP DIVE

> *"Transformation is often more about unlearning than learning."*
> – **Richard Rohr**

Awakening to the idea that one can explore and find the root cause of PMDD symptoms is a transformative realization. Traditional approaches, while providing tremendous relief and playing a crucial role in managing symptoms, often act as temporary solutions. These methods can ease our journey but rarely address the underlying issues. When we start connecting the dots between our emotional symptoms and the luteal phase, we uncover a profound link between unmet needs, unresolved pain, and our subconscious mind. This revelation serves as a powerful reminder that our emotions and physical symptoms are not random occurrences; they are deeply rooted in the subconscious patterns formed during our early years. Understanding this connection is a pivotal step in our holistic path to healing PMDD, guiding us toward a journey of deeper reflection and self-awareness. As we seek relief and freedom from PMDD, it becomes clear that true liberation comes from an inward journey—one that only you can take for yourself. This awakened journey calls us to be the heroes of our own stories, empowering us to find the strength and wisdom within to truly set ourselves free.

This is exactly where my journey began, and looking back, I could not believe I did not know this earlier. Despite years of conversations with medical professionals, therapists, and counselors, I had never encountered this life-changing information. But when I discovered and came to understand that there is work that can get to the root cause, everything began to make sense. I realized that for as long as I could remember, I had believed there was something fundamentally wrong with me. I thought I was flawed, broken, and beyond repair. I convinced myself that I was created this way, perhaps cursed and that this was the thorn in my side, the cross I had to bear, the best that God had for me. I believed I was destined to endure this deep, relentless pain throughout my life.

In high school, I distinctly remember the dark place that seemed to consume me. No matter how hard I tried to surface for air, it would pull me back under, time and time again. To think that I lived this way for over 25 years is almost unimaginable; I do not know how I survived. But now, as I begin to understand the pain and my story, it all starts to make sense. I realize that my journey was meant to bring me to this point.

My deepest hope and desire are that you cling to these words and embark on your own journey of inner work and self-discovery. May you find encouragement and light in knowing that you do not have to suffer and that you were not made to endure this kind of pain. You were meant to understand it, to understand yourself, and to break free from the prison that has held you captive. Your pain has a purpose, and that purpose is to lead you to a place of healing and self-awareness, where you can finally set yourself free, becoming you, truly you.

The more I explored and researched the subconscious mind, the clearer it became that emotional pain was at the core of my symptoms. And when I began to do the work, what surprised me were all the small, seemingly insignificant moments from my childhood that left lasting imprints on me and in me. Moments I was told to brush off, times that I was told to get over it but couldn't—instances where I felt hurt, ashamed, unloved, not heard, or alone— formed the foundation of my belief system. The memories I shared when I was six years old— it was these events along with others; it was the "minor" hurts and experiences and the misinterpretations that I made about them that shaped my thoughts and beliefs about myself.

Through the deep work I have done, I have uncovered suppressed memories and feelings and recognized their impact on my life. A fleeting childhood moment that led to a negative feeling can evolve into a persistent belief, creating an operating system that governs our actions and self-perception. Understanding this was transformative for me. It revealed how my subconscious mind was driving my PMDD and all my symptoms, allowing me to address these beliefs and heal from them.

It was these moments that led to a negative feeling that evolved into a persistent belief, creating an operating system that governed my feelings and self-perception. Understanding this was transformative for me. It revealed how my subconscious mind was driving my PMDD and all of my symptoms, allowing me to re-address these moments while still validating my experiences, viewing them now as an adult, releasing those feelings, and changing my beliefs is where I began to heal from them.

The incredible workings of our mind hold the key to understanding how our beliefs shape our reality and influence every aspect of our lives. As children, we were simply trying to understand our surroundings and ourselves, crafting thoughts, interpretations, feelings, and beliefs. As adults now, whatever we experience, our brains process these past moments, drawing the meaning influenced by our past encounters, emotions, and pre-existing beliefs.

Consider this: if, as a child, you were reprimanded for sharing your thoughts, you might have felt shame or embarrassment. This emotional imprint can embed itself deep within your subconscious, creating a belief that speaking out is harmful or unwelcome. Over time, this belief directs your thoughts, emotions, and actions.

This process forms a feedback loop: a negative experience sparks a strong emotional reaction, which then solidifies into a belief. This belief then shapes later emotions and thoughts, influencing future behaviors. For example, if you believe that sharing your opinions is wrong, you might habitually hold back in conversations, further cementing the original belief and its associated emotional response.

Such interpretations can mistakenly transform an isolated incident into a perceived universal truth, establishing false beliefs. These beliefs can become deeply entrenched, influencing our reactions to similar events across our lives, affecting our self-esteem, social interactions, and overall health.

The repercussions on our physical health are significant. Holding onto negative beliefs can cause chronic stress or tension, as our nervous system treats these beliefs like constant threats, supporting a perpetual state of vigilance. This can manifest physically as headaches, muscle tension, digestive problems, and even chronic ailments.

These beliefs also influence our behavior. For instance, if we believe we are undeserving of love, we might inadvertently push others away or undermine our relationships, thus perpetuating a cycle of loneliness and isolation. Our thoughts, molded by these beliefs, turn into self-fulfilling prophecies. Expecting rejection, our actions unconsciously mirror this belief, often leading to the very rejection we anticipate.

Understanding the formation and impact of these beliefs is crucial for healing. By bringing these subconscious beliefs to light, we can begin to question their validity and replace them with healthier, more accurate perceptions of ourselves and the world. This process involves deep introspection, often through practices like therapy, meditation, or journaling, where we can safely explore our inner world and uncover the root causes of our pain.

Ultimately, the journey to healing involves recognizing the incredible power of our mind to shape our reality. By addressing and transforming our false beliefs, we can change our thoughts, feelings, behaviors, and even our physical health, paving the way for a more fulfilling and authentic life.

THE WORKINGS OF OUR BRAINS

Neuroplasticity is the brain's remarkable ability to reorganize itself by forming new neural connections throughout life. This means our brains are not static; they can change and adapt based on our experiences, thoughts, and behaviors. When we consistently think or act in a certain way, our brain strengthens the neural pathways associated with those patterns. Conversely, when we stop engaging in a particular thought or behavior, those neural connections weaken. This adaptability is what allows us to change deeply ingrained beliefs and habits.

The subconscious mind plays a pivotal role in this process. Unlike the conscious mind, which processes information actively and deliberately, the subconscious mind works below the surface, influencing our thoughts, feelings, and behaviors without us even being aware of it. It stores all our memories, experiences, and learned behaviors, shaping our automatic responses to various situations.

When a belief becomes ingrained in our subconscious, it can feel like an undeniable truth, even if it is based on a misinterpretation or a singular event from our past. These subconscious beliefs form the core of our self-perception and worldview, driving our automatic reactions and decisions. Because the subconscious mind is so powerful, changing these ingrained beliefs requires consistent and deliberate effort.

OUR GREATEST ALLY

Neuroplasticity is one of our greatest allies in healing, offering the ability to rewire the brain by challenging and reframing false beliefs. By consistently practicing affirmations, positive self-talk, and intentional behavioral changes, we can create new neural pathways that support healthier and more empowering perspectives. Over time, these pathways become deeply ingrained in the subconscious, reshaping how we think, feel, and respond to life's challenges.

This remarkable adaptability of the brain allows us to move beyond limiting beliefs and emotional patterns that have held us back. Neuroplasticity is not just about change—it is about transformation. It gives us the power to rewrite our inner narratives, enabling profound improvements in mental and emotional well-being. For me, discovering a therapy that uses these science-based approaches to uncover and address deep-seated causes of pain was absolutely life-changing. This approach not only allowed me to heal but also offered a path to lasting transformation, proving that we all have the potential to rewire our minds and reshape our lives.

RTT

Rapid Transformational Therapy, or RTT, is a therapeutic approach that stands out for its deep and immediate impact on emotional and psychological issues. Developed by Marisa Peer, RTT combines elements from various therapeutic methods to offer a unique and powerful tool for healing. This therapy is not just about talking over problems; it is about transforming lives from the roots.

Marisa Peer is an internationally acclaimed hypnotherapist with advanced qualifications from the Hypnotism Training Institute of Los Angeles. She holds certifications in hypno-healing, advanced hypnotherapy, medical hypnotherapy, and Gestalt analysis. Additionally, Marisa has furthered her expertise through studies at the Proudfoot School of Hypnotherapy and Psychotherapy and the Atkinson Ball College of Hypnotherapy.

With over three decades dedicated to the meticulous research, testing, and application of the most effective principles of hypnotherapy, psychotherapy, NLP, CBT, and neuroscience, Marisa has developed a distinctive approach known as Rapid Transformational Therapy® (RTT). This unique method has transformed the lives of tens of thousands of individuals worldwide, helping them to overcome personal challenges and achieve greater happiness and fulfillment.

Marisa is also a best-selling author of six books, translated into multiple languages, and a prominent columnist and contributor to publications such as Closer and Men's Fitness, as well as major Sunday newspapers.

She frequently appears as an expert on the BBC and other global television networks. Recognized for her impact, Marisa was featured in The Midas List: 22 Successful British Women to Follow in 2022. She has been invited to speak at prestigious events, including TEDx, Condé Nast, and the Royal Society of Medicine, sharing her passionate and effective approach to transforming lives from within.

RTT is built on the understanding that many mental and emotional struggles, including PMDD, are rooted in past experiences and subconscious beliefs often formed in childhood. These deeply ingrained patterns shape how we think, feel, and react as adults. RTT does not just analyze these beliefs—it transforms them. By diving into the subconscious mind through hypnosis, RTT uncovers and addresses the root causes of these challenges, initiating profound change.

What sets RTT apart is its focused and integrative approach, blending the principles of Hypnotherapy, Cognitive Behavioral Therapy (CBT), and Neuroscience. Using hypnosis as a gateway, clients are guided into a relaxed yet heightened state of awareness, where the conscious mind steps aside, allowing the subconscious to become highly receptive to positive change. This process leverages the brain's neuroplasticity—the ability to adapt and rewire itself—helping clients reshape their thoughts and behaviors by addressing deep-seated memories and beliefs.

RTT does not just look to fix what feels broken; it reveals and enhances the beauty and strength already within you. Imagine peeling back layers of outdated beliefs and fears, uncovering the true essence of who you are, untouched by the struggles of the past. This transformative journey is about rewriting your life's narrative, shifting from limitation to empowerment, and discovering a new way of being—free, whole, and resilient.

As you reflect on RTT, consider this: How might uncovering the root causes of your challenges and rewriting your inner story transform the way you live and thrive? Let's explore further.

THE CORE COMPONENTS OF RTT

Rapid Transformational Therapy (RTT) is a powerful, integrative approach to healing that combines hypnotherapy, cognitive-behavioral therapy (CBT), and neuroscience, particularly neuroplasticity. Hypnotherapy serves as a gateway to the subconscious, uncovering deeply ingrained beliefs and emotional patterns, while CBT helps reframe negative thought processes into healthier, more constructive ones.

Neuroplasticity—the brain's natural ability to rewire itself—enhances RTT's transformative power by replacing limiting beliefs with empowering ones. Techniques like guided regression and personalized recordings reinforce these changes, creating new neural pathways for lasting growth. By harmonizing these elements, RTT fosters profound emotional and psychological transformation, offering a comprehensive pathway to personal well-being and resilience.

HYPNOTHERAPY: UNLOCKING THE SUBCONSCIOUS

Hypnotherapy, a cornerstone of Rapid Transformational Therapy (RTT), is a powerful and scientifically grounded technique designed to create meaningful and lasting change. Often misunderstood as mystical, hypnotherapy is a well-documented process that guides individuals into a deeply relaxed, focused state. This state, akin to a meditative or trance-like experience, is something we naturally experience like becoming engrossed in a book or movie and losing track of time. During this state, the brain shifts from active beta waves to slower alpha or theta waves, associated with relaxation, creativity, and heightened receptivity.

What makes hypnotherapy transformative is its ability to bypass the critical, analytical mind and access the subconscious—the part of the mind where deeply rooted memories, beliefs, and emotional patterns reside. The subconscious operates like the software of a computer, running the programs that shape our behaviors and feelings. Many of these "programs" are formed in early life and continue to influence us, often without our conscious awareness, even if they no longer serve us.

Through hypnotherapy, RTT practitioners uncover and address the root causes of emotional and psychological challenges stored in the subconscious. This process allows for the identification and removal of harmful "viruses" like negative beliefs and traumas and the installation of positive "updates" such as empowering life-affirming beliefs. By reprogramming the mind's internal scripts, hypnotherapy fosters healthier emotional and psychological functioning.

Far from being mystical or magical, hypnotherapy uses the brain's natural adaptability to promote profound healing. It taps into the foundation of thought and behavior, allowing individuals to reshape their inner narratives and achieve lasting transformation. By working directly with the subconscious, RTT uses hypnotherapy to unlock the mind's potential, creating a pathway for personal growth, emotional freedom, and a more fulfilling life.

ADDRESSING MYTHS AND MISCONCEPTIONS

Despite its scientific basis, hypnotherapy is often surrounded by myths and misconceptions. Here are some common myths and the scientific truths behind them:

1. **Myth: Hypnotherapy is Mind Control.**
   - **Truth**: Hypnotherapy does not involve controlling someone's mind or making them do things against their will. In reality, individuals are fully aware and in control during the session. They can choose to accept or reject any suggestions made by the therapist.

2. **Myth: You Can Get Stuck in Hypnosis.**
   - **Truth**: It is impossible to get stuck in a hypnotic state. If a session were to end abruptly, a person would naturally return to full awareness on their own, much like waking from a daydream.

3. **Myth: Hypnotherapy is Just Relaxation.**
   - **Truth**: While relaxation is a component, hypnotherapy goes much deeper, targeting the subconscious mind to address and resolve deep-seated issues. It is not merely about feeling calm but about making profound and lasting changes.

4. **Myth: Hypnotherapy is Unscientific.**
   - **Truth**: Hypnotherapy is backed by a substantial body of scientific research. Studies have shown its effectiveness in treating various conditions, from anxiety and depression to chronic pain and PTSD. It works by altering brain wave patterns and increasing neuroplasticity, which enhances the brain's ability to change and adapt.

REGRESSION THERAPY

Regression therapy is a key part of RTT. In regression therapy, you revisit past experiences that have significantly shaped how you think, feel, and react today. This process is not about lingering in the past but rather about understanding and reinterpreting those experiences to foster healing and enable forward movement.

Taking a moment for reflection: think about an experience that continues to affect your emotions or behavior negatively month after month. How might viewing this experience through a new lens change its impact on you? Reflect on how re-interpreting this memory could support you in your healing. What would it feel like to release the weight of that experience and replace it with understanding, compassion, or empowerment?

PART WORKS THERAPY

As we come to the final pages of this journey, let us reflect on the metamorphosis of the butterfly—a symbol of profound transformation and renewal. The caterpillar, content yet confined, represents the beginning of our journey, living within the limitations of pain, patterns, and the familiar. But deep within, there is a call to something greater, an unshakable knowing that change is possible. The cocoon, though dark and isolating, mirrors the sacred, uncomfortable process of healing—a time to face shadows, release what no longer serves, and surrender to the unknown. Finally, as the butterfly emerges, wings glistening with new colors, it reminds us of the beauty and freedom that come from embracing our highest selves. For those with PMDD, this transformation is a testament to the courage it takes to shed the old and embody a life of balance, self-love, and purpose. Your healing is your rebirth; may you soar, light and free, into the radiant future you were always meant to live.

CBT AND INNER CHILD HEALING

RTT incorporates Cognitive Behavioral Therapy (CBT) to help identify and reframe negative thought patterns that influence their emotions and behaviors. By exploring the subconscious mind, the session helps pinpoint the root causes of these beliefs and uses techniques inspired by CBT to challenge and replace them with healthier, empowering thoughts. This enables a shift in perspective, breaking free from self-limiting cycles.

INNER CHILD HEALING

Inner child healing is a transformative process that addresses unresolved emotional wounds and unmet needs from childhood. Rooted in the understanding that our early experiences significantly shape our beliefs, behaviors, and emotional responses, this approach focuses on reconnecting with the "inner child"—a subconscious part of us that keeps the emotions and memories of our formative years. Negative or traumatic childhood experiences often leave lasting impressions, influencing our mental and emotional well-being well into adulthood.

The healing journey begins by acknowledging and validating the pain and emotions tied to those early experiences. Techniques such as visualization and dialogue help foster compassion for the inner child, allowing individuals to reconnect with and understand their younger selves. A crucial step is reparenting, where one provides the love, care, and support that was lacking in childhood. This nurtures a sense of safety and fulfills unmet needs, releasing stored emotional pain and trauma.

Central to this process is transforming negative beliefs born from childhood experiences, such as feeling unworthy or unsafe, and replacing them with empowering truths. As healing progresses, individuals begin to view these past experiences through their adult eyes, recognizing that they are no longer living in that moment or bound by those feelings. This integration process brings freedom from the recurring emotional responses rooted in childhood, allowing for greater emotional stability and healthier patterns of thought and behavior.

The impact of inner child healing is profound. It leads to improved self-esteem, healthier relationships, and a deeper sense of peace and fulfillment. By nurturing and reparenting the inner child, individuals achieve lasting transformation, breaking free from the past and embracing a more empowered and authentic life.

THE SCIENCE AND SOUL BEHIND RTT

Rapid Transformational Therapy (RTT) uses the science of neuroplasticity—the brain's ability to rewire itself—to address the root causes of Premenstrual Dysphoric Disorder (PMDD). During RTT sessions, clients uncover deep-seated beliefs and traumas through guided regression therapy. After these sessions, therapists create personalized audio recordings filled with positive, affirming suggestions tailored to the client's specific needs. By listening to these recordings daily for 21 to 30 days, clients engage their brain's neuroplasticity, reinforcing new, empowering beliefs, and forming new neural pathways. This consistent practice replaces old, limiting patterns with healthier ones, leading to profound and lasting transformation.

WHERE SCIENCE MEETS SOUL

This process beautifully illustrates the convergence of science and soul. The scientific principles of neuroplasticity provide a foundation for tangible change, allowing individuals to actively reshape their brains and, so, their lives. On a deeper level, RTT touches the soul by healing emotional wounds and reconnecting individuals with their true selves. It honors the human spirit's capacity for growth and aligns neurological change with personal and spiritual development. By integrating cutting-edge neuroscience with profound inner healing, RTT offers a holistic approach that not only alleviates PMDD symptoms but also fosters a renewed sense of wholeness, fulfillment, and authentic living.

NEUROLOGICAL CHANGES

RTT leverages the brain's natural adaptability to address the root neurological causes of PMDD. By reprogramming neural pathways through tailored techniques, it reduces emotional swings and stabilizes stress responses, promoting a sense of balance and relief from PMDD's challenges. This transformation not only alleviates symptoms but also empowers individuals to embrace a more peaceful and fulfilling life.

RTT also focuses on reshaping emotional responses by engaging the subconscious mind, uncovering, and rewriting the deep-seated narratives that amplify PMDD symptoms. This process not only relieves immediate distress but also builds long-term emotional resilience. As you reflect on the shifts RTT can bring, consider how altering these subconscious patterns aligns with your spiritual growth and personal aspirations. The ability to rewire your brain highlights your innate ability for healing, inspiring a journey toward greater inner peace and alignment with your highest self.

ENHANCING NEUROLOGICAL AND EMOTIONAL INTEGRATION

Rapid Transformational Therapy (RTT) facilitates profound, lasting change by embedding healthier patterns of thinking and emotional regulation into your daily life. Through consistent reinforcement, these changes become second nature, transforming your responses and behaviors in a sustainable and practical way. This reprogramming helps prevent the recurrence of severe PMDD symptoms, fostering a more stable and fulfilling life. Personalized recordings play a vital role in this process, replacing old, limiting beliefs with empowering ones that align with your true self.

As these changes take root, they reflect a broader journey of healing—one that bridges the mind, body, and spirit. RTT does not just address PMDD; it invites you to explore the interconnectedness of your inner world, opening the door to profound transformation. This journey allows you to live more authentically, aligning your actions and aspirations with your deepest values.

The number of RTT sessions needed for PMDD varies depending on individual circumstances, emotional resilience, and symptom complexity. Most individuals experience significant change within one to three sessions, though added sessions may be beneficial to fully address all aspects of the condition. Follow-up sessions can help reinforce progress, address emerging issues, and support the integration of new beliefs and behaviors.

RTT's effectiveness is grounded in both science and countless personal stories of transformation. It respects the complexities of the brain and the depth of the human spirit, offering a therapeutic path that inspires hope and real change. By trusting in the process, you embrace the potential for healing and open yourself to new possibilities for a balanced, fulfilling, and empowered life.

A TOOL FOR GROWTH

RTT is more than just a method for healing; it is a tool for profound personal growth. Imagine a life without PMDD—what would it be like? Truly, what would it be like for you? Imagine waking up each day free from the shadow of your severe emotional and physical symptoms. Envision engaging in your daily activities with a newfound sense of calm and resilience. Feel the lightness in your body, the clarity in your mind, and the peace in your spirit. Your family and personal relationships flourish as you communicate with openness and understanding, no longer hindered by the emotional turbulence of PMDD. Your professional life thrives as you focus and perform without the recurring disruptions of your condition. Personal pursuits and passions reignite, allowing you to explore and enjoy life's offerings with enthusiasm and joy. Being free from PMDD feels like reclaiming your life and stepping into a version of yourself that radiates confidence, self-love, and compassion...becoming YOU again.

As you wrap up this chapter, take a moment to truly envision your transformation. There is a pathway to reclaim your true self. This healing journey is not just about mitigating symptoms; it is about awakening to a new reality where you are empowered, balanced, and aligned with your highest potential. Imagine stepping into this new life with confidence, knowing that you have the tools and the support to sustain this transformation. Let this vision inspire you as you continue your path to healing and personal growth.

INTRODUCTION TO CASE STUDIES AND THE IMPACT OF RTT

I wanted to provide a deeper look at the transformative experiences of PMDD clients who took part in my Living in Luteal Programs, exploring the profound impact of Rapid Transformational Therapy on their lives. Each client engaged in one of the three different program options: private sessions, group support, and self-led study. These case studies illustrate how these approaches to healing from PMDD can lead to significant and lasting change.

THE LIVING IN LUTEAL PROGRAM

The Living in Luteal Program is designed to address the unique challenges of PMDD by focusing on the luteal phase of the menstrual cycle. This program offers three distinct pathways to cater to unique needs and preferences:

1. **Private Sessions**: One-on-one RTT sessions tailored to the individual's specific experiences and challenges, providing personalized support and deep healing.
2. **Group Support**: A community-based approach where participants benefit from shared experiences, weekly support calls, and collective healing guided by RTT principles.
3. **Self-Led Study**: A flexible, self-paced program that includes guided RTT sessions, educational materials, and transformational recordings to empower individuals to take charge of their healing journey.

TRANSFORMATIVE JOURNEYS: PRIVATE PROGRAM

The Living in Luteal Private Program is a comprehensive healing and transformative journey tailored to address the deep-rooted causes of PMDD. This chapter delves into compelling case studies, showcasing the remarkable transformations experienced by individuals from various occupations. Through three RTT sessions, weekly support, and daily listening to transformational recordings, each participant found profound healing and freedom from PMDD.

Case Study 1: A Film Producer's Path to Peace

Background: Sophia, a successful film producer, was grappling with severe anxiety and panic attacks. Her volatile emotions led to frequent fights with her partner, straining their relationship. The pressure of her high-stakes career compounded her stress, making her PMDD symptoms unbearable.

Journey: Sophia's journey through the Living in Luteal program began with intense RTT sessions that uncovered deep-seated fears and unresolved traumas from her past. These fears were driving her anxiety and emotional volatility. By addressing these root causes, Sophia started to dismantle the patterns that were exacerbating her PMDD.

The program's weekly support calls provided Sophia with strategies to manage her stress and maintain emotional stability. Daily listening to her personalized transformational recordings reinforced her new beliefs, promoting a sense of inner peace and resilience.

Outcome: By the end of the program, Sophia had healed the root cause of her PMDD symptoms. She is now free from anxiety and panic attacks, and her relationship with her partner has improved dramatically. Sophia navigates her career with newfound confidence and emotional balance, living a life of peace and fulfillment.

Case Study 2: A Photographer's Journey to Freedom

Background: Michelle, a talented photographer, found herself unable to leave his house due to crippling anxiety and depression. Her career was in jeopardy, and her relationship was suffering as she withdrew further into isolation during her luteal phase.

Journey: Michelle's RTT sessions revealed underlying beliefs of inadequacy and fear of judgment rooted in childhood experiences. These beliefs were paralyzing her and contributing to her severe PMDD symptoms. Through the program, Michelle began to reframe these beliefs and build a healthier self-image.

Weekly support calls offered Michelle practical advice and emotional support, helping her gradually regain her confidence. Her daily transformational recordings played a crucial role in solidifying these new, empowering beliefs.

Outcome: By the end of the program, Michelle had overcome the root causes of her PMDD. He is now able to leave her house and engage with her passion for photography. Her relationship has improved, and her career is back on track. Michelle experiences the luteal phase with stability and optimism, living a life of freedom and creativity.

Case Study 3: An Executive's Return to Harmony

Background: Jessica, a high-level executive, struggled to balance her demanding career, home life, and marriage. PMDD symptoms left her feeling overwhelmed and incapable of managing her responsibilities, leading to conflicts at work and home.

Journey: Jessica's RTT sessions uncovered deep-rooted feelings of guilt and pressure to be perfect, stemming from her upbringing. These feelings were driving her PMDD symptoms and creating chaos in her life. By addressing these issues, Jessica began to reclaim her sense of control and self-worth.

The weekly support calls taught her techniques for managing her stress and prioritizing her well-being. Her daily transformational recordings reinforced her new beliefs, fostering a sense of balance and harmony.

Outcome: By the end of the program, Jessica had healed the root cause of her PMDD symptoms. She now manages her career with confidence, keeps a harmonious home life, and enjoys a fulfilling marriage. Jessica is PMDD-free and navigates the luteal phase with grace and composure.

Case Study 4: A College Student's Journey to Hope

Background: Ava, a college student and aspiring artist, was struggling with suicidal thoughts and hopelessness. Her PMDD symptoms made it impossible to handle her academic tasks and pursue her creative passions, leaving her feeling lost and desperate.

Journey: Ava's RTT sessions revealed profound feelings of unworthiness and fear of failure rooted in her past experiences. These feelings were fueling her PMDD symptoms and driving her to despair. Through the program, Ava began to heal these wounds and build a stronger sense of self-worth.

Weekly support calls offered Ava emotional support and practical strategies to manage her studies and creative pursuits. Her daily transformational recordings helped rewire her brain, instilling hope, and resilience.

Outcome: By the end of the program, Ava had found the root cause of her PMDD symptoms and experienced a remarkable transformation. She is now PMDD-free, feeling hopeful and inspired. Ava handles her academic tasks with confidence and pursues her artistic passions with renewed vigor. She has embraced a life of balance and creativity.

TRANSFORMATIVE JOURNEYS: GROUP PROGRAM

The Living in Luteal program for PMDD offers a holistic journey designed to address the root causes of Premenstrual Dysphoric Disorder through a combination of Rapid Transformational Therapy (RTT), weekly support calls, and daily transformational recordings. This chapter explores three deeply personal and inspiring case studies, highlighting the transformative power of this program.

Case Study 1: A Single Mom's Path to Stability

Background: Sarah, a single mom of two young children, was constantly struggling to make ends meet. The relentless demands of balancing work and family, coupled with the debilitating symptoms of PMDD, left her feeling overwhelmed and hopeless. Her mood swings, intense irritability, and severe anxiety during the luteal phase of her menstrual cycle were affecting her ability to provide for her family and keep a sense of stability.

Journey: Sarah embarked on the Living in Luteal program with a mix of hope and skepticism. Her RTT sessions unearthed deep-seated beliefs of inadequacy and fear of failure, stemming from a childhood marked by instability and criticism. Through guided regression, Sarah was able to confront these beliefs and begin the process of reshaping her self-perception.

The weekly support calls provided a safe space for Sarah to share her experiences, receive encouragement, and learn from others in similar situations. Listening to her transformational recordings daily reinforced the new, empowering beliefs she was cultivating.

Outcome: By the end of the four-month program, Sarah had found the root cause of her PMDD symptoms. She experienced a profound shift in her emotional and mental state, leading to a significant reduction in her PMDD symptoms. Sarah is now PMDD-free, living a life of balance and confidence. She has secured a stable job, providing a nurturing environment for her children, and navigates the luteal phase with newfound resilience and peace.

Case Study 2: An Artist's Journey to Self-Discovery

Background: Emily, a talented freelance artist, and member of Alcoholics Anonymous (AA), had been battling PMDD alongside her recovery from alcohol addiction. The intense emotional upheaval during her luteal phase worsened her feelings of self-doubt and insecurity, threatening her sobriety and stifling her creative expression.

Journey: The Living in Luteal program offered Emily a comprehensive approach to addressing her PMDD. In her RTT sessions, Emily uncovered unresolved grief and trauma related to her past struggles with addiction and the loss of a close family member. This understanding allowed her to release the emotional pain she had been carrying.

The program's weekly support calls were instrumental in Emily's progress. The sense of community and mutual support reinforced her commitment to both her recovery and her healing journey. Daily listening to her transformational recordings helped rewire her brain, fostering a sense of self-worth and stability.

Outcome: Emily emerged from the program, having found the root cause of her PMDD symptoms. She is now PMDD-free and thriving as an artist. Her creative work has flourished, and she maintains her sobriety with greater ease. Emily's luteal phase is no longer a period of turmoil but one of balanced creativity and inner peace.

Case Study 3: A Mother of Four's Return to Harmony

Background: Heather, a mother of four, was at her wit's end. The relentless demands of parenting, coupled with the debilitating effects of PMDD, left her feeling disconnected and overwhelmed. Her severe mood swings and depressive episodes during the luteal phase strained her relationship with her children and husband, creating a chaotic home environment.

Journey: Heather joined the Living in Luteal program, seeking relief and a way to reconnect with her family. Her RTT sessions revealed deep-rooted feelings of guilt and self-sacrifice linked to her upbringing and the pressures of motherhood. Confronting these emotions allowed Hannah to begin healing and redefining her sense of self.

The weekly support calls provided Heather with invaluable insights and practical advice on managing her symptoms and nurturing her relationships. The daily practice of listening to her transformational recordings reinforced her new beliefs, promoting a sense of balance and self-compassion.

Outcome: By the end of the program, Heather had uncovered the root cause of her PMDD symptoms and achieved a remarkable transformation. She is now PMDD-free, experiencing harmony and joy in her daily life. Her relationship with her children and husband has significantly improved, and she navigates the luteal phase with confidence and emotional stability.

TRANSFORMATIVE JOURNEYS: SELF-GUIDED PROGRAM

The Living in Luteal Self-Guided Program offers a powerful, independent approach to addressing the root causes of Premenstrual Dysphoric Disorder (PMDD). Utilizing pre-recorded RTT sessions and hypnosis recordings, participants embark on a journey of self-reflection and inward renewal. This chapter explores three compelling case studies that highlight the significant relief and transformation achieved through this self-led program.

Case Study 1: A School Teacher's Journey to Stability

Background: Amy, a dedicated schoolteacher and single mom, was struggling to manage her responsibilities due to the severe emotional and physical symptoms of PMDD. Her mood swings, irritability, and fatigue during the luteal phase were affecting her performance at work and her ability to care for her children.

Journey: Amy enrolled in the Living in Luteal Self-Guided Program with a sense of urgency and hope. Through the pre-recorded RTT sessions, Amy explored the deep-seated beliefs and unresolved emotional issues that were contributing to her PMDD symptoms. The hypnosis recordings provided her with daily reinforcement of new, positive beliefs and coping mechanisms.

The work guide led Amy through an inward journey of self-reflection and renewal. She journaled her thoughts and feelings, gaining insights into her triggers and patterns. This process helped her build a stronger connection with herself and her needs.

Outcome: By the end of the program, Amy experienced significant relief from her PMDD symptoms. She became more emotionally stable and less reactive, both at work and at home. Emily now navigates the luteal phase with greater ease and confidence, allowing her to perform effectively as a teacher and be a more present and patient mother.

Case Study 2: A Single Mom's Path to Empowerment

Background: Hannah, a single mom of two, was overwhelmed by the demands of raising her children while battling PMDD. The intense mood swings, anxiety, and depression during her luteal phase left her feeling exhausted and unable to fully engage with her children or her own needs.

Journey: Hannah turned to the Living in Luteal Self-Guided Program, seeking a lifeline. The pre-recorded RTT sessions helped her uncover and address the root causes of her emotional turmoil. Through hypnosis recordings, Hannah reinforced new, empowering beliefs daily, which gradually replaced her old, limiting patterns.

The work guide helped Hannah's journey of inward reflection. She used journaling to delve into her experiences and emotions, uncovering insights that led to greater self-awareness and understanding.

Outcome: By the conclusion of the program, Hannah had achieved a remarkable transformation. She found significant relief from her PMDD symptoms, feeling more balanced and in control of her emotions. Hannah's newfound stability allowed her to better manage the demands of single parenthood, fostering a more harmonious and nurturing environment for her children.

Case Study 3: A Path to Renewal After Job Loss

Background: Catherine, a dedicated professional, lost her job due to the debilitating effects of PMDD. Her severe mood swings, depression, and lack of focus during the luteal phase made it impossible for her to keep up her performance at work, leading to her eventual dismissal.

Journey: Desperate for a solution, Jane enrolled in the Living in Luteal Self-Guided Program. The pre-recorded RTT sessions guided her to the core issues underlying her PMDD symptoms, helping her to confront and heal from past traumas and negative beliefs. Daily hypnosis recordings reinforced these positive changes, promoting a sense of calm and resilience.

Using the work guide, Catherine embarked on a journey of self-reflection and renewal. She journaled extensively, gaining clarity on her triggers and emotional patterns. This process empowered her to rebuild her self-confidence and sense of purpose.

Outcome: By the end of the program, Catherine had experienced profound relief from her PMDD symptoms. She regained emotional stability and clarity, which allowed her to seek new employment with renewed confidence. Jane now approaches her luteal phase with a sense of balance and control, and she has secured a new job where she excels, free from the limitations previously imposed by PMDD.

LONG TERM POST RTT: A PERSONAL TESTIMONY

While much of the support for Rapid Transformational Therapy currently relies on case studies and client experiences, there is an increasing effort to confirm its effectiveness through more robust scientific research. Early clinical trials and systematic reviews are starting to examine the full scope of RTT's impact, particularly its long-term effects on patients. Yet, beyond this growing body of scientific evidence, I serve as living proof of the deep and lasting transformations RTT can create.

MY JOURNEY TO FREEDOM

For years, I lived in the shadow of Premenstrual Dysphoric Disorder—a relentless cycle that consumed every part of me. The emotional volatility, crippling anxiety, and soul-crushing depression that came with each luteal phase left me feeling trapped and powerless. PMDD did not just affect my body; it infiltrated my mind, my relationships, and my sense of self. My personal life was in shambles, my family life was strained, and my professional world felt impossible to sustain. I was barely holding it together, clinging to whatever scraps of normalcy I could find.

I will admit that when I first came across RTT, I was skeptical. After years of failed attempts to find relief, I was not sure anything could help me—but I was desperate. I began my journey with RTT cautiously, yet something inside me whispered to keep going. What I discovered during those sessions was profound. Through guided regression, I faced the deep-seated beliefs and emotional pain I had buried for so long. It was an intensely emotional experience but one of the most validating moments of my life. For the first time, I was able to see my experiences through my adult eyes and realize how deeply my feelings and responses were linked to little Rachel—still in pain, still connected to the past, and still needing to heal.

It became clear that the wounds I had carried for so long were begging to be mended. RTT gave me the tools to do that. The personalized recordings I listened to daily became more than just words—they were the affirmations I had longed to hear as a child—that I am lovable, I am loved, I am safe, I am worthy, and I am enough. Slowly, as I listened to these words' day after day, they began to rewire my brain. The neural pathways that once carried pain and doubt were replaced with pathways of love, safety, and self-worth. What once felt impossible became my new belief system.

Today, I stand here PMDD-free. The mood swings, anxiety, and depression that once ruled my life are gone. I have reclaimed my sense of self-worth, confidence, and peace—things I once believed were out of reach. My home is now a place of love and laughter, my relationships have deepened, and my professional life is thriving in ways I never thought possible. I now move through my luteal phases with balance and ease, something I could only dream of before.

This is not just a story about RTT—it is my story, my transformation. RTT did not just help me heal; it gave me the power to rewrite the narrative of my life. The changes I have experienced are not fleeting; they have fundamentally reshaped how I live, how I love, and how I see myself. RTT gave me my life back, and for that, I am endlessly grateful.

A CRY FOR HOLISTIC INCLUSION: ADVOCATING IN A PHARMACEUTICAL-DRIVEN HEALTHCARE SYSTEM

Researching treatments for PMDD can be both enlightening and disheartening. Major medical resources often focus on pharmaceutical solutions like SSRIs and hormonal therapies, while holistic approaches—including transformative therapies like Rapid Transformational Therapy (RTT)—are notably absent from mainstream recommendations. This raises a critical question: why are potentially effective and science-backed therapies not part of the broader conversation?

The omission of therapies like RTT, often dismissed as "woo-woo," reflects a deeper issue in healthcare—one rooted in fear, bias, and profit-driven motivations. By prioritizing pharmaceutical interventions over comprehensive care models, the system risks limiting sufferers' access to holistic solutions that address the root causes of conditions like PMDD. This narrow focus leaves many individuals feeling unseen and unsupported despite their need for deeper healing. This is not just a matter of medical preference; it is a profound issue of justice. Every woman has the right to be informed of all available treatment options, not just those that are traditionally endorsed.

Holistic approaches, which encompass RTT, mindfulness, nutrition, neuroscience, and psychotherapy, are not just alternatives—they are integral to a more inclusive and effective treatment model. It is not a matter of rejecting traditional medicine but of expanding the spectrum of care to include therapies that treat the whole person: mind, body, and spirit. The lack of such options in mainstream discourse underscores a pressing need for education, advocacy, and systemic change.

True healing requires a balanced, informed approach. By embracing therapies like RTT alongside traditional treatments, we can offer PMDD sufferers the comprehensive care they deserve—care that moves beyond symptom management to empower lasting transformation and hope.

THE PATH FORWARD

As the scientific community continues to validate Rapid Transformational Therapy, my journey stands as living proof of its profound impact. I, along with others who no longer suffer from PMDD, am a testament to the deep inner work RTT provides. This therapy does not just offer temporary relief—it delivers life-changing transformation, helping individuals heal at their core.

Through RTT, I have not only alleviated my PMDD symptoms but also reconnected with my true self, experiencing a level of freedom and wholeness I never thought possible. My story is shared with the hope of inspiring others to believe in their own ability for healing. The path to lasting change may be challenging, but it is within reach. With the powerful tools of RTT and the courage to embark on this journey, you, too, can create a life of balance, peace, and true transformation.

The message of hope I share is rooted in the belief that healing, freedom, and even a cure from PMDD are truly possible. My own journey led me to Rapid Transformational Therapy (RTT), a powerful modality that helped me uncover and address the root cause of my emotional pain. RTT is an incredible tool that has proven to be effective in treating PMDD by working with the subconscious mind and promoting inner healing. However, while I am a voice of hope and deeply believe in the possibility of healing, I want to empower you to explore what resonates with your unique journey. There are other approaches involving trauma healing, neuroplasticity, and subconscious work that can significantly support your path. Healing is personal, and while RTT was the path that worked for me, it may not be the only way. I encourage you to trust yourself as you uncover what leads you to true wholeness and healing.

Chapter Nine

YOUR HIGHER IDENTITY & SELF IS CALLING

> *The Higher Self is whispering to you softly in the silence between your thoughts.*
> **-Deepak Chopra**

PMDD is like experiencing identity theft once a month, as it profoundly impacts a person's sense of self and emotional stability. Just as identity theft takes away control of one's identity, PMDD can make a woman feel like their true selves are overtaken by an unrecognizable version. It steals the essence of who you are—your purpose, your truth, your light, your hope, your gifts, your sensitivity, and your calling. In those dark moments, it can feel like the real you is buried beneath layers of pain, depression, anxiety, and anger. But what if I told you that your most healed and whole self is calling to you, always urging you to reclaim your authenticity, gifts, sensitivity, and light? It is time to step into the life you deserve and are worthy of having.

THE CALL TO RECLAIM YOUR IDENTITY

PMDD is not just a disorder; it is a thief of your unique identity. Each month, it takes away bits and pieces of who you are, leaving you feeling disconnected and lost. But deep within, your true self remains, waiting to be rediscovered. Healing from PMDD is not just about alleviating symptoms; it is about reclaiming your identity and stepping into your highest self.

AWAKENING YOUR TRUE SELF

As you step into this healing journey, a new world starts to reveal itself—a world where pain, anxiety, and anger no longer define you. You may find yourself asking, "Who am I without the pain? What will life feel like without depression, anxiety, or constant irritation?" These questions are natural as you step into the unknown, exploring peace and wholeness for the first time. Healing from PMDD becomes a deep and intimate journey of letting go of everything you are not, to embracing everything that you are and who you have truly come here to be.

Although these thoughts may seem unusual, it is often the fear of the unknown that keeps us stuck in old patterns. But what I have learned is that everything we desire lies just beyond fear. By taking the leap, you open the door to a new inner reality that begins to shape your outer world as well.

Imagine navigating your luteal phase grounded in who you are, self-understanding, compassion, and overall balance. Each day becomes something to embrace, free from the shadows PMDD has cast over your life. Your whole and healed self is not a far-off dream but a true reality waiting for you once you release the hold of those gripping shadows and fully step into your authentic self.

THE JOURNEY BEYOND PAIN

Your most authentic or highest self refers to the deepest, truest version of oneself, unencumbered by societal expectations, fears, and past traumas. This concept is about recognizing and embracing the core of who you are at your most positive, peaceful, and empowered. Here are some key aspects of the highest self:

1. **True Nature:** Your highest self is the essence of who you really are, your fundamental nature that exists beyond the roles, masks, and identities that are often imposed by the outside world.
2. **Inner Wisdom:** It represents a state of being where you are deeply connected to your intuition and inner wisdom. This is the part of you that knows what is best for you and guides you towards actions and decisions that align with your true purpose and happiness.
3. **Unconditional Love:** Your highest self embodies unconditional love and acceptance, not only for others but also for yourself. It fosters a compassionate outlook, allowing you to see and accept your flaws and virtues alike.
4. **Peace and Composure:** This aspect of you remains calm and centered, even in the face of challenges and chaos. It brings a sense of peace that does not waver with external circumstances.
5. **Freedom from Limiting Beliefs:** Living as your highest self involves shedding limiting beliefs and fears that hinder your growth and happiness. It is about transcending the doubts that keep you from embracing your full potential.
6. **Connectedness**: Your highest self understands the interconnectedness of all life and experiences a profound sense of unity with others and the universe. This awareness fosters empathy and a strong sense of belonging.
7. **Joy and Fulfillment**: Operating from your highest self leads to genuine joy and fulfillment because you are living in alignment with your deepest values and desires. It means engaging with life authentically and passionately.

Recognizing and nurturing your highest self is a process that encourages not just personal happiness and success but also a meaningful contribution to the world around you.

EMBRACING YOUR NEW REALITY

Now, imagine your healed, authentic self emerging during each luteal phase—stepping into your true power and essence, free from the shadows of PMDD.

As this version of you awakens, your luteal phase becomes a time of introspection and deep self-awareness rather than turmoil. Each month, instead of feeling overwhelmed by emotions, you experience clarity and insight. You begin to notice that your body and mind are speaking to you, revealing hidden truths, but without the overwhelming weight of anxiety or anger.

Physically, your body feels lighter. The tension and fatigue that once drained your energy is replaced by a sense of grounded strength. Your movements are more fluid, your posture more confident, and you feel in tune with your body's rhythms. There is a quiet energy within you that is calm yet powerful, helping you navigate this phase with grace.

Emotionally, you feel centered. Instead of being swept away by irritability or sadness, you are able to observe your emotions without being controlled by them. You can acknowledge any discomfort with compassion, understanding that it is part of a deeper healing process. The overwhelming sense of peace you now feel allows you to respond to triggers thoughtfully rather than reacting impulsively.

Mentally, your thoughts are clearer. The fog that once clouded your mind during this phase has lifted, and you are able to focus, think creatively, and make decisions without second-guessing yourself. You trust your intuition more, knowing that it is guiding you toward what truly aligns with your soul's purpose.

Spiritually, you feel connected to something greater. You are more in tune with your inner wisdom and sense of purpose, seeing the luteal phase as a sacred time for self-reflection and growth. Instead of resisting this phase, you welcome it as a time to nurture yourself and realign with your highest values.

In this state, you feel empowered to embrace each day, knowing that your authentic self is becoming stronger, more balanced, and more in harmony with who you are meant to be. The luteal phase no longer feels like a burden—it becomes a portal to deeper healing, transformation, and self-love.

During this journey, you learn to establish better personal boundaries. You discover that you have a voice and that your feelings are safe. This newfound confidence transforms your relationships. Marriages are restored as you and your partner communicate more openly and empathetically. Your bond with your children strengthens as you become more present, understanding, and supportive.

You become the cycle breaker, ending the generational trauma that has been passed down. By doing so, you not only heal yourself but also pave the way for a healthier, more harmonious family dynamic. You become the trailblazer of healing in your home and family, a beacon of light and hope. Healing is not just a personal experience; it creates a ripple effect, touching the lives of those around you and spreading positivity and transformation.

As you embrace this, you become a living testament to the power of healing and growth. Your journey inspires others to seek their own paths to wellness, creating a community of support and understanding. The changes you make within yourself extend outward, influencing the world in profound and meaningful ways. You embody the essence of resilience and hope, illuminating the way for others to follow.

STEPPING INTO YOUR LIGHT

Your highest self is calling you to step into your light and embrace the life you deserve. This journey is about more than just surviving PMDD; it is about thriving well beyond it. As you continue to heal, you will find that your true self is not defined by the struggles you faced but by the strength and wisdom you have gained through them.

REFLECTION QUESTIONS

1. What aspects of your identity have you felt disconnected from due to PMDD?

   _____

   _____

   _____

2. How does the idea of reclaiming your true self resonate with you?

   _____

   _____

   _____

3. What are some gifts and talents you have rediscovered or want to explore as you heal?

_____

_____

_____

4. How can you nurture your emerging self during this period of adjustment?

_____

_____

_____

5. What does stepping into your highest authentic self look like for you, what would that feel like for you?

_____

_____

_____

As you respond, let it stir something within you—a cry, a call, as deep calls to deep, an awakening to redeem your true infinite and endless worth. You are not defined by PMDD; you are not defined by your symptoms. You are defined by the light within you, the truth of who you are, and the gifts you have to offer the world. The life you yearn for, ache for, and deserve is within you. Answer the call. Reclaim your identity. Embrace your light. Embrace your truth. It is time.

The very intent of God, Source, higher intelligence, or the universe—whatever name you choose to resonate with—was that you were created whole, complete, and boundless, with infinite potential and a purpose that transcends limitations. You were designed to live without restrictions, without a ceiling to your growth, expansion, or capabilities. Consider for a moment the essence of a baby, how they exist in their purest state—curious, joyful, and constantly learning. They move through life with open hearts and open minds, fully present in each moment.

From the moment you entered this world, you carried within you a divine spark—a unique essence, a blueprint for your greatness that no one else possesses. This personal code, your potential, was woven into the fabric of your being before you ever took your first breath. As infants, we naturally express the truest form of our existence, encountering the world with a sense of awe and wonder. Whether it is feeling the warmth of the sun on our skin or hearing the soothing voice of someone we love, we engage fully, with an eagerness to discover the beauty around us.

In this state of purity, we are untainted by fear, doubt, or limitation. Each new experience is met with excitement and a thirst for learning because our souls are wired for growth and expansion. This drive within us—the urge to explore, create, and understand—is the manifestation of the divine intention that we should live in fullness, never confined by the boundaries of the world or our own minds.

As we grow, many of us begin to lose touch with this pure, limitless nature. Life, with its challenges and pressures, often leads us to build walls around ourselves, disconnecting from that original state of boundless potential. We may adopt beliefs about limitations, adopt fears about failure, and create glass ceilings where none were ever meant to exist.

But that divine spark, that infinite potential, never truly leaves us. It remains within, waiting to be reawakened. Reclaiming that truth means remembering that you were never meant to be small, to be restricted, or to live beneath your potential. You were created to flourish, to explore life with the same wonder you once did as a child, to expand without limitation, and to realize that the only barriers in life are the ones we allow ourselves to believe in.

By reconnecting with your essence, you begin to break down those glass ceilings. You remember that you were created with the purpose of living fully— experiencing love, growth, creativity, and joy in abundance. The very foundation of your existence is divine, limitless, and worthy of everything you desire and more. This is the truth of who you are, and it is always within you, waiting to be embraced and fully expressed.

Our growth never stops. Consider nature; a seed planted in the earth contains all the potential to become a towering tree. It grows, adapts, and flourishes, reaching for the sky without restraint. Similarly, we are meant to continuously evolve, uncovering our true selves, and aligning with our highest purpose.

In the same way, our personal and spiritual growth is an ongoing journey. We are constantly evolving, shaped by our experiences and the wisdom we gain along the way. Every challenge we face, and every lesson we learn contributes to our development, pushing us closer to our true selves. This process is not linear; it involves moments of struggle and breakthrough, much like the tree enduring harsh weather yet standing tall and firm.

This divine blueprint for growth is echoed in the scriptures. Jeremiah 29:11 reassures us of God's plans for our prosperity and well-being, promising hope and a future. Psalm 139:14 celebrates our unique creation, affirming that we are "fearfully and wonderfully made." Philippians 4:13 empowers us with the strength to overcome challenges through divine support. These verses collectively underscore the belief that we are designed for continuous growth and fulfillment.

Aligning with our highest purpose requires us to shed limiting beliefs and embrace the fullness of our potential. It calls for a return to this childlike state of wonder and curiosity, approaching life with an open heart and mind. By doing so, we tap into the limitless possibilities that exist within us, breaking free from the confines of fear and doubt.

These insights guide us on our spiritual journey towards a deeper understanding of our place in the universe. They encourage us to align our actions with our divine purpose, seek healing, and embrace the infinite possibilities that lie ahead. By grounding ourselves in these spiritual truths, we can navigate life's challenges with a sense of peace, purpose, and profound joy. Our journey of growth and self-discovery is a sacred one, deeply intertwined with the divine plan for our lives. Embracing this truth allows us to live authentically and joyously, aligned with the divine purpose that resides within us.

SPIRITUAL LAWS AND HIGHER SELF

The idea of the higher self is prominent in many spiritual teachings and philosophies. It is often associated with the understanding that we are more than just our physical bodies and minds. Spiritual laws, such as the Law of Attraction, suggest that our thoughts, feelings, and intentions are powerful forces that shape our reality. Aligning with our higher self means tuning into these spiritual laws and understanding that we are co-creators of our existence.

THE LAW OF ATTRACTION

The Law of Attraction is one of the most recognized spiritual laws, embodying the adage that "like attracts like." This principle suggests that the energy and thoughts we emit into the universe attract similar energies and outcomes back to us. This means that positive thoughts and intentions can attract positive experiences and opportunities, while negative thoughts and feelings can attract negative experiences.

DEEPER EXPLANATION OF THE LAW OF ATTRACTION

The Law of Attraction is rooted in the belief that our thoughts have a tangible, energetic power. Each thought generates a specific energy that can interact with the universe on a similar frequency. When you think positively, you emit high-frequency energy, which attracts circumstances that also resonate at high frequencies, such as joy, peace, and success.

Conversely, negative thoughts emit a lower frequency and can attract negative circumstances, such as conflict, sadness, and obstacles. The process is not just about thinking something and expecting it to appear; it involves a deeper connection with the subconscious mind. It is believed that our subconscious mind influences the energy we emit, which shapes our experiences and reality. By aligning our conscious and subconscious thoughts with what we desire, we create a powerful force that makes manifestation possible.

Key Aspects of the Law of Attraction

1. Intention Setting: Clear intentions provide a roadmap for the universe to respond to. By setting specific, positive intentions, you clarify what you wish to attract, making it easier for the universe to deliver.
2. Visualization: Imagining the desired outcome in detail can enhance manifestation. This practice involves mentally picturing yourself in the scenario you wish to manifest, complete with emotional and sensory details.
3. Affirmations: These are positive, present-tense statements that reinforce your ability to manifest your desires. Regularly reciting affirmations can help reshape your thoughts and energy, aligning them with your goals.

4. Gratitude: Keeping a grateful attitude boosts your frequency and enhances your ability to attract more of what you are thankful for. Gratitude shifts your focus from what you lack to what you have, which is essential for manifesting abundance.

5. Persistence and Belief: Confidence in the process and persistence in your practices are crucial. Doubt can introduce negative energy that hampers the manifestation process.

6. Alignment and Action: While the Law of Attraction emphasizes the power of thoughts and feelings, aligned actions are necessary to realize your intentions.

POWER OF AFFIRMING YOUR HIGHEST SELF AND PURPOSE

Affirming your highest self and your highest purpose taps deeply into the Law of Attraction by aligning your everyday actions and choices with your ultimate values and aspirations. When you affirm your highest self, you acknowledge and strive to realize your fullest potential. This practice involves recognizing your intrinsic worth, your capabilities, and your right to personal growth and fulfillment.

By focusing on your highest purpose, you send a powerful message to the universe about your intentions. This not only attracts the experiences and resources you need to fulfill your purpose but also aligns your personal energy with the energy of your aspirations. Such alignment enhances your overall well-being, as it brings coherence between your inner desires and your external life, fostering a sense of peace, satisfaction, and fulfillment. Utilizing the Law of Attraction to affirm your highest self involves regularly visualizing yourself as the person you aspire to be, employing affirmations that reflect your deepest values and goals, and expressing gratitude for the journey and its lessons.

BIBLICAL PRINCIPLES AND HIGHER SELF

From a biblical perspective, the higher self can be equated with the concept of the "new man" or the "spirit-filled life" mentioned in the New Testament. Verses such as Ephesians 4:22-24 urge believers to put off the old self and put on the new self, created to be like God in true righteousness and holiness. This transformation is seen as a journey towards becoming more Christ-like, having a Christ-consciousness, embodying virtues like love, compassion, and humility.

The scriptures also provide profound insight into the power of the mind and its profound influence on our lives. As Romans 12:2 exhorts, "but be transformed by the renewing of your mind," it highlights the transformative potential that comes from nurturing and renewing our mental landscapes. This process of transformation is not merely about changing how we think but is about fundamentally altering our inner being to align more closely with our divine purpose and true self.

Proverbs 23:7 says, "For as he thinketh in his heart, so is he," reminding us that our deepest thoughts and beliefs shape who we are and what we become. This verse underscores the idea that our identity and actions are a reflection of our inner thoughts and convictions, pointing to the importance of cultivating a mindset that supports our highest aspirations.

This sets the stage for understanding the rules of how your mind works, emphasizing the importance of actively shaping our thoughts to reflect our true selves.

Here are some essential rules that illustrate how our minds work, guiding us towards personal transformation and the realization of our highest potential:

10 EASY RULES TO UNDERSTAND HOW THE MIND WORKS

1. The Mind Adheres to What It Focuses On: Our mind tends to bring about what it dwells on. Focusing on negative aspects can reinforce limiting beliefs, while focusing on positive possibilities can pave the way for empowerment.
2. Beliefs Shape Perception: Our beliefs act as lenses through which we view the world. They shape our perceptions and can either limit or expand our view of possibilities.
3. Thoughts Trigger Emotions: Every thought generates a corresponding emotion. Negative thoughts trigger negative emotions, sustaining a cycle of self-limiting patterns.
4. The Mind Seeks Confirmation: Through confirmation bias, our mind looks for information that supports our existing beliefs. This can reinforce limiting beliefs unless consciously challenged.
5. Habitual Thinking Patterns Rule: Much of our thinking is habitual. These automatic thought patterns dictate our default reactions and behaviors.

6. Emotions Influence Decisions: Our emotions can drive our decisions more powerfully than logic. This can keep us tethered to limiting beliefs unless we develop emotional awareness and regulation.
7. Repetition Reinforces Pathways: Neuroplasticity shows that repeated thoughts and behaviors strengthen neural pathways, making repeated patterns more dominant over time.
8. The Subconscious Stores Beliefs: Many of our beliefs are stored in the subconscious, influencing our behavior without our conscious awareness.
9. Visualization Can Change Outcomes: Imagining a different outcome can reprogram the mind to make it more receptive to change and new possibilities.
10. The Mind Can Be Rewired: With consistent effort and techniques such as mindfulness, meditation, and cognitive restructuring, it is possible to change our mental wiring and adopt new, empowering beliefs.

Embracing both the spiritual perspective and the rules of the mind offers a holistic approach to personal transformation, guiding us to live out our truth and achieve our true potential through the deliberate renewal and nurturing of our thoughts.

THE ROAD TO EVOLVING AND ASCENSION

The journey towards aligning with our higher self is an ongoing process involving continuous self-reflection, growth, and transformation. As we evolve, we shed layers of limited beliefs and ego-driven behaviors, moving closer to our most authentic and healed selves. This process is often described as a spiritual ascent, where we gradually raise our consciousness and vibrational frequency.

Continuous Growth

Continuous growth is the cornerstone of spiritual evolution. It demands an unwavering commitment to self-improvement and a willingness to confront and release outdated patterns and beliefs. This journey is marked by:

- **Self-Reflection**: Regular introspection helps us identify areas where we are not aligned with our higher self. By examining our thoughts, feelings, and actions, we can pinpoint limiting beliefs and ego-driven behaviors that need to be transformed.

- ✧ **Personal Development**: Engaging in practices that promote personal growth—such as reading, learning new skills, and seeking mentorship—enables us to expand our horizons and enhance our understanding of ourselves and the world.
- ✧ **Spiritual Practices**: Meditation, mindfulness, and other spiritual practices facilitate a deeper connection with our inner self and the divine. These practices help raise our vibrational frequency and align us with our true purpose.
- ✧ **Emotional Healing**: Addressing and healing past traumas is crucial for shedding layers of the ego. This process often involves therapy, self-compassion, and forgiveness, allowing us to release emotional baggage and move forward with greater clarity and peace.

MANIFESTATION

Manifestation is the process of bringing our beliefs, desires, and intentions into physical reality, and it begins with the thoughts and emotions we hold about ourselves. Whether we realize it or not, what manifests in our lives is a reflection of our inner world—our belief system about who we are and what we deserve. For those suffering from PMDD, this becomes particularly significant, as the symptoms they experience often manifest from deeper emotional and mental patterns, acting like a self-fulfilling prophecy.

When our beliefs are rooted in fear, self-doubt, or negative self-worth, those beliefs manifest as chaos in our lives, reinforcing the idea that we are somehow broken, unworthy, or defined by pain. PMDD sufferers may feel trapped in cycles of depression, anxiety, and anger, leading them to believe that these emotions are part of their identity when, in truth, they are symptoms of deeper, unresolved patterns.

However, the same energy that brings painful manifestations can be redirected to serve our highest good. By recognizing that our experiences are a mirror of our inner world, we can shift our beliefs and, in turn, transform our manifestations. This is how we move from living in a state of reactivity and survival to a state of intention and creation, aligning our lives with our highest purpose and potential.

Manifesting from a Place of Limitation:

Imagine a PMDD sufferer who believes, deep down, that she is powerless over her emotions. Every month, she expects PMDD to take over her life. Her belief system is dominated by thoughts like, *"I'm not strong enough to handle this,"* or *"I'm always going to suffer like this."* These thoughts, repeated over time, begin to shape her reality. She starts to notice that each time her luteal phase begins, her mood darkens, and the smallest stressors trigger anxiety, depression, or rage. This becomes her lived experience, reinforcing her belief that she has no control. In this way, her thoughts, and beliefs about herself create a manifestation of pain and struggle, locking her in a cycle of suffering.

Manifesting from a Place of Empowerment:

Now consider a PMDD sufferer who has chosen to believe that healing is possible. Instead of viewing her condition as something that defines her, she views it as an opportunity to deepen her self-awareness and grow. Her thoughts shift from *"I am broken"* to *"I am healing and learning more about myself each day."* She begins to focus on what brings her peace and balance during her luteal phase, whether it is practicing mindfulness, nurturing her body with healthy foods, or setting boundaries that honor her emotional needs. By aligning her actions with the belief that she has the power to influence her experience, she begins to manifest more positive outcomes—less emotional volatility, more self-compassion, and greater inner peace. Her belief system now works in harmony with her desires, allowing her to create a life that reflects her healing rather than her pain.

Key Aspects of Positive Manifestation:

1. **Clarity of Intentions**: The first step in manifestation is defining what we truly want. For someone with PMDD, this might look like setting an intention for peace and emotional stability rather than being consumed by the anticipation of symptoms. When we are clear about our desires, we can direct our energy toward them, shaping our actions and thoughts in alignment with those goals.

   Example: "I intend to experience calm and resilience in my luteal phase." This intention, if held with clarity, begins to shape behaviors—like prioritizing self-care and practicing emotional awareness—that support that outcome.

2. **Positive Mindset**: Our mindset plays a crucial role in what we manifest. If we believe we are victims of our circumstances, we will continue to experience life as such. However, if we keep a mindset of growth and empowerment, we attract experiences that support our evolution.

   Example: A PMDD sufferer who shifts from, *"I hate this time of the month, I always suffer,"* to *"This time teaches me how to nurture myself more deeply"* will begin to experience her luteal phase as a time for self-discovery rather than dread.

3. **Aligned Actions**: Manifestation is not passive. It requires us to take purposeful and consistent actions that align with our desires. A PMDD sufferer who wants to heal must take daily steps that support her well-being, whether that is through nutrition, rest, therapy, or other healing modalities.

   Example: If the desire is to feel balanced emotionally, aligned actions could include implementing a daily meditation practice, setting boundaries to reduce stress, or seeking professional support.

4. **Gratitude**: Gratitude amplifies the energy of manifestation. By focusing on what is going right in our lives and being thankful for progress, no matter how small, we signal to the universe that we are ready to receive more of that positive energy.

   Example: A PMDD sufferer who expresses gratitude for the days when she feels good or for the strength, she shows even on difficult days is likely to attract more moments of peace and resilience. Gratitude helps to shift the focus from suffering to healing, from scarcity to abundance.

Transforming Negative Manifestations:

When we recognize that the painful experiences, we endure are often the result of underlying limiting beliefs, we can start the process of transformation. Instead of unconsciously allowing our fears or negative self-perceptions to shape our reality, we can consciously choose to adopt beliefs that serve our highest good. This means rewiring the inner dialogue from thoughts of *"I can't handle this,"* to *"I am capable of healing and transforming my experience."*

By doing so, we convert the experience of suffering into an opportunity for growth. Rather than seeing PMDD as an obstacle, it becomes a tool for self-discovery, teaching us to listen to our bodies, nurture our minds, and align with our true, highest selves. In this way, the manifestation process becomes a way to move from pain to purpose, from survival to thriving. What once felt like a curse can transform into a path toward self-empowerment, where you can live fully in your power, unburdened by past limitations.

THE SCIENCE OF LIGHT: QUANTUM PHYSICS AND NEUROSCIENCE

As we delve into the fascinating overlap of spirituality and science, we uncover a profound truth: we are, in the most literal sense, beings of light. Did you know that at the moment of conception, a remarkable event occurs: a spark of light is generated? This phenomenon, both symbolic and scientific, represents the beginning of new life, where the fusion of sperm and egg creates a burst of energy, signifying the start of a unique human existence.

Quantum physics has revealed that at the most fundamental level, we are composed of particles of light—photons. This scientific revelation beautifully aligns with spiritual teachings, particularly the concept of being light bearers. In Matthew 5:14, it is written, "You are the light of the world." Amazing right?!

This statement, once purely spiritual, now finds resonance in the realm of science, affirming the intrinsic light within each of us. Quantum physics tells us that these photons are not just particles but also waves of energy that hold information. This dual nature of light echoes the duality of our existence: we are both physical and spiritual beings. The energy we emit and absorb shapes our reality, suggesting that our thoughts, emotions, and intentions can influence the world around us. This idea is a cornerstone of many spiritual practices, which advocate for the power of positive thinking, intention setting, and mindfulness.

Neuroscience further enriches this understanding by shedding light on the remarkable capabilities of the human brain. The concept of neuroplasticity has revolutionized our understanding of the brain's potential.

Dr. Joe Dispenza, a renowned neuroscientist and author, has extensively explored the transformative power of the mind. He states, "The brain is the organ of change. When you change your mind, your brain literally changes, and when your brain changes, you change your life". This highlights the incredible potential we have to shape our destinies through conscious thought and intention. By changing our patterns of thinking, we can rewire our brains, leading to significant shifts in our behavior, emotions, and overall well-being.

From a spiritual perspective, this ability to change and grow is seen as a divine gift. It reflects the belief that we are created in the image of God, endowed with the capacity for limitless growth and transformation. The alignment of scientific discoveries with spiritual teachings offers a holistic view of our existence, where science validates and deepens our understanding of ancient spiritual wisdom.

The intersection of quantum physics, neuroscience, and spiritual wisdom offers a profound insight: we are beings of light, equipped with the natural capacity to reshape our lives through the power of our minds. This understanding encourages us to step into our full potential, tap into the energy of our thoughts, and actively shape the reality we experience. It is an invitation to awaken to our true essence, realizing that we embody both the light of the universe and the creators of our own paths.

ONGOING JOURNEY

Our journey to our higher self is never-ending, revealing new layers of potential and deeper truths with each step. The empowerment and truth we gain fuel our continued evolution, requiring us to adapt, grow, and expand our consciousness. By embracing this ongoing journey, we align more closely with our higher self, experiencing greater fulfillment and alignment with our divine purpose. As we heal, evolve, and ascend, we transform not only our own lives but also contribute to the collective elevation of human consciousness, bringing us closer to the divine essence within us. This journey is a call to awaken our true nature, recognizing that we are both the light of the world and the architects of our own destinies.

This book is not the end but a beginning—a starting point for a deeper exploration into your health and spiritual life, as well as your menstrual, mental, and emotional well-being. As you continue to apply these principles, remember that growth is a continuous journey. There will be setbacks and breakthroughs, but each step brings you closer to a fuller understanding of yourself and your potential.

May this book serve as a guiding light, reminding you that you hold the power to shape your health and happiness. Embrace each day with a sense of determination, seeing it as a chance to strengthen your resilience and nurture joy. Your journey through PMDD is uniquely your own, and within it lies the opportunity for deep personal growth and transformation. Keep learning, exploring, and evolving—your path is filled with infinite possibilities.

A CALL TO REMEMBRANCE

May you remember who you truly are. Beneath the layers of conditioning, past experiences, and external expectations, there exists an original blueprint—your unique personal code, intricately woven into the very fabric of your being. This code, embedded in your cells and your energetic framework, holds the key to your highest potential and the truest expression of your soul.

To remember is not simply to recall a distant memory but to tap into the essence of your divine design, that which has been present within you from the moment of creation. Spiritually, this remembrance is a reconnection to the deeper wisdom of your soul, the part of you that has always known your purpose, your path, and your limitless capacity for growth. It is awakening to the truth that you were created intentionally, with a purpose that is written into every fiber of your being.

Science, too, supports this idea. Quantum physics and neuroscience teach us that our bodies and minds are dynamic systems deeply interconnected with the energy of the universe. Every cell in your body carries the imprint of your unique identity and potential. The neurons in your brain form pathways that mirror your beliefs and thoughts, shaping your reality. To remember is to tap into this synergy between spirit and science, recognizing that you are not separate from the greater whole but an integral part of the cosmic design.

This remembrance is an act of empowerment, allowing you to reclaim the parts of yourself that have been lost or forgotten along the way. As you reconnect with your original blueprint, you begin to realize that the answers you seek have always been within you. You are capable of profound healing, growth, and transformation because your personal code has been designed for exactly that.

May you awaken to this remembrance daily, embracing both the spiritual and scientific truths that affirm your potential. In doing so, you will walk the path of your highest self, guided by the wisdom that has always been yours.

THE AWAKENED ACTION

My prayer is that through the pages of this book, you are awakening, opening, and feeling the connection within. I hope this message resonates deeply with you and leads you on a path to self-discovery and healing.

I want to give you a way to begin this transformative work, a roadmap to begin your next step forward that guides you through each step of your journey. That is why I created RESTORE, a self-care luteal phase guide designed to support you in this awakened journey towards truth and light. The simple workbook and the meditations that are included are your starting guide on this brave new path, helping you to navigate the complexities of PMDD with compassion and understanding.

As a free gift to you, I invite you to begin your journey with RESTORE. This is an opportunity to embrace an awakened and mindful approach to PMDD, empowering you to take the first steps towards profound personal transformation.

WHAT IS RESTORE?

RESTORE embodies an awakened and mindful approach to managing PMDD, offering a structured yet flexible framework to guide you through your healing process. Let's explore a sneak peek glance at each element in detail:

RECOGNIZE: ACKNOWLEDGE THE IMPACT

The first step in your journey is to RECOGNIZE the profound impact PMDD has on your life. This means acknowledging the physical, emotional, and psychological toll it takes. By being honest with yourself about your experiences, you create a foundation for genuine healing. This recognition is not about dwelling on the pain but about understanding its presence and preparing to address it with compassion.

EXPLORE: INVESTIGATE SUBCONSCIOUS ELEMENTS

Next, EXPLORE the subconscious elements contributing to your emotional pain and triggers. This involves delving into the hidden parts of your psyche, where past traumas and unresolved emotions reside. Through meditation, journaling, and mindful reflection, uncover these buried elements. Exploring these areas allows you to understand the roots of your suffering, making it possible to heal from within.

SEE: REASSESS PAST EXPERIENCES

With newfound insights, SEE your past experiences from a mature, understanding perspective. This step is about reassessing the stories you have told yourself and the beliefs you have formed. By seeing these experiences with clarity and wisdom, you can release old patterns and begin to rewrite your narrative. This process helps you to let go of what no longer serves you and opens the door to healing.

TRANSFORM: APPLY NEW INSIGHTS

Now, it is time to TRANSFORM. Apply the insights gained from your exploration and reassessment to shift your relationship with PMDD. This transformation is both internal and external. Internally, it involves changing your thought patterns and emotional responses. Externally, it might mean altering your lifestyle, seeking new forms of support, or adopting healthier habits. Transformation is an ongoing process, but with each step, you move closer to a life of balance and peace.

OVERCOME: REPLACE NEGATIVE BELIEFS

To OVERCOME, you must replace negative beliefs with empowering affirmations. Negative self-talk and limiting beliefs can keep you trapped in a cycle of suffering. By consciously choosing to affirm your worth, strength, and resilience, you begin to dismantle these barriers. Overcoming is about empowering yourself with positivity and self-love, reinforcing the belief that you can thrive despite PMDD.

RECONNECT: HEAL EMOTIONAL WOUNDS

RECONNECT with your inner child to heal emotional wounds. This step is about nurturing the parts of yourself that have been hurt and neglected. By reconnecting with your inner child, you offer comfort, understanding, and unconditional love. This reconnection helps to mend emotional wounds and fosters a sense of wholeness and self-acceptance.

EMPOWER: EQUIP YOURSELF

Finally, EMPOWER yourself with strategies for better emotional management and well-being. This includes practical tools such as stress reduction techniques, healthy lifestyle choices, and building a supportive community. Empowerment is about taking control of your health and well-being and equipping yourself with the knowledge and resources needed to navigate life's challenges with grace and resilience.

EMBRACING YOUR HEALING JOURNEY

This journey is not a linear path but one of continuous growth and self-discovery. Each cycle, each phase, brings new insights and opportunities for healing. Embrace the cyclical nature of your journey, allowing yourself the grace to move at your own pace.

As we come to the final pages of this journey, let us reflect on the metamorphosis of the butterfly—a symbol of profound transformation and renewal. The caterpillar, content yet confined, represents the beginning of our journey, living within the limitations of pain, patterns, and the familiar. But deep within, there is a call to something greater, an unshakable knowing that change is possible. The cocoon, though dark and isolating, mirrors the sacred, uncomfortable process of healing—a time to face shadows, release what no longer serves, and surrender to the unknown. Finally, as the butterfly emerges, wings glistening with new colors, it reminds us of the beauty and freedom that come from embracing our highest selves. For those with PMDD, this transformation is a testament to the courage it takes to shed the old and embody a life of balance, self-love, and purpose. Your healing is your rebirth; may you soar, light and free, into the radiant future you were always meant to live.

A JOURNEY TO THE LIGHT

As you embark on this journey of healing and self-discovery, remember that you are not alone. Countless individuals are walking this path with you, reclaiming their power, and embracing their true selves. Together, we are creating a new narrative, one where menstrual and mental health is understood, honored, and celebrated.

Your journey to the light is a testament to your strength, resilience, and unwavering spirit. Embrace each step with compassion and love for yourself. Trust in your body's wisdom and the transformative power of healing. You are worthy of this journey, and the light that awaits you reflects the beauty and power within you.

In the words of the great poet Rumi, *"The wound is the place where the Light enters you."* May your journey be filled with light, love, and endless possibilities.

This now marks the end of this book but the beginning of your personal journey into healing. Take the RESTORE process to heart and let it guide you toward a life of balance, empowerment, and profound self-awareness. You have the tools, the knowledge, and the strength to transform your relationship with PMDD and step into the light of your true self. I see *you*.

**Sending you much love, sending you much light—
I love you, Rachel**

FROM CURSED TO CURED

RESTORE.

An awakened & mindful approach to PMDD

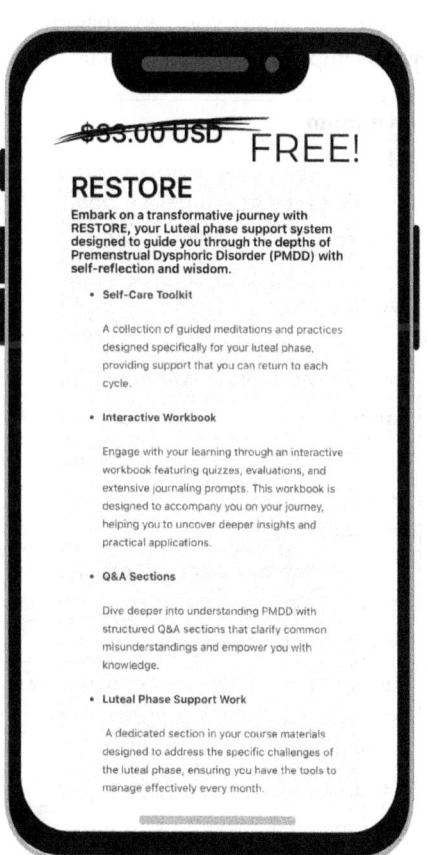

Discover a journey of healing and growth with RESTORE, your Luteal phase support system designed to guide you through the complexities of PMDD with self-reflection and wisdom.

This course offers an opportunity to awaken to your fullest potential by empowering you to manage and understand your symptoms not just as a challenge, but as a pathway to profound personal growth.

Through guided meditations, practical tools, and reflective journaling, RESTORE helps you turn your luteal phase into a time of healing and self-discovery, fostering a deeper connection with yourself and your emotional well-being. This is your beginning, your first steps into the world of inner work and self-awareness.

Experience RESTORE for FREE!

Visit: www.rachellynnfox.com/offers/H5DhPXnU?coupon_code=RESTORE100 to start your free journey of healing and growth, self-reflection, and wisdom.

PMDD Luteal Phase Self-Assessment Tool

Instructions: Rate each symptom below based on your experiences during the luteal phase (the period between ovulation and the start of menstruation). Use a scale from 0 to 10, where 0 means no symptoms, and 10 means the most severe symptoms you can imagine. This will allow you to better understand your symptoms in order to facilitate a discussion with your healthcare provider.

Symptom	0	1	2	3	4	5	6	7	8	9	10
Mood Swings											
Sudden or intense shifts in mood, such as from happiness to sadness or anger.											
Depression											
Feelings of hopelessness, worthlessness, or persistent sadness.											
Anxiety											
Excessive worry, tension, or feeling on edge.											
Irritability											
Easily annoyed or angered, often with little provocation.											
Sensitivity to Rejection											
Feeling overly sensitive to criticism or perceived rejection, leading to emotional distress.											
Fatigue											
Extreme tiredness or lack of energy, even after adequate rest.											
Sleep Disturbances											
Difficulty falling asleep, staying asleep, or waking up feeling unrefreshed.											
Physical Symptoms											
Bloating, breast tenderness, headaches, joint or muscle pain.											
Appetite Changes											

Increased cravings, overeating, or loss of appetite.								
Concentration Issues								
Difficulty focusing, remembering, or making decisions.								

TOTAL SCORE:

After rating each symptom, add up your scores to get a total. This will help you and your healthcare provider understand the severity of your PMDD symptoms during the luteal phase.

- 0-20: Mild Symptoms
- 21-40: Moderate Symptoms
- 41-60: Severe Symptoms
- 61-80: Very Severe Symptoms
- 81-100: Extremely Severe Symptoms

Take a moment to reflect on your scores.

Are there any symptoms that stand out as particularly challenging?

_____

_____

_____

How do these symptoms impact your daily life and relationships?

_____

_____

_____

Use this tool as a starting point for discussions with your healthcare provider about your PMDD management for traditional and holistic treatment options.

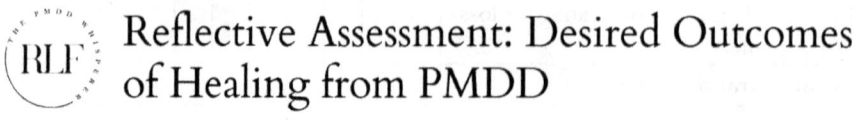 Reflective Assessment: Desired Outcomes of Healing from PMDD

This reflective assessment is designed to help you connect with your deepest desires for healing and envision the positive changes that can come from no longer living with PMDD. Keep this as a guide and reminder of your goals and aspirations as you continue your healing journey.

Instructions:

- Before answering these questions, take a moment of reflection and engage in a 5-minute moment of silence in prayer or meditation. Connect with the most healed version of yourself that already exists.
- Reflect on your answers deeply, envisioning a life without PMDD.

Emotional Well-Being:

Question: How would your emotional well-being change if you no longer experienced PMDD?

Answer: _____

_____

_____

_____

Personal Relationships:

Question: How would your relationships with your husband, partner, children, friends, and loved ones improve?

Answer: _____

_____

_____

_____

Self-Esteem and Confidence:

Question: How would your self-esteem and confidence be affected by the absence of PMDD symptoms?

Answer: _____

_____

_____

_____

Work or School Performance:

Question: What changes would you see in your ability to perform at work or school?

Answer: _____

_____

_____

_____

Physical Health:

Question: How would your physical health and energy levels improve?

Answer: _____

_____

_____

_____

Social Life:

Question: How would your social life and ability to engage in activities you enjoy change?

Answer: _____

_____

_____

_____

Mental Clarity and Focus:

Question: How would your mental clarity and ability to concentrate be affected?

Answer: _____

_____

_____

_____

Stress and Anxiety Levels:

Question: How would your levels of stress and anxiety change?

Answer: _____

_____

_____

_____

Sleep Quality:

Question: What improvements would you see in your sleep quality and patterns?

Answer: _____

_____

_____

_____

Financial Stability:

Question: How would your financial situation improve, and how would your work performance shift?

Answer: _____

_____

_____

_____

Life Goals and Aspirations:

Question: How would achieving a life without PMDD impact your pursuit of life goals and aspirations?

Answer: _____

_____

_____

_____

Personal Growth and Development:

Question: How would your personal growth and development be enhanced?

Answer: _____

_____

_____

_____

Daily Responsibilities:

Question: How would your ability to manage daily responsibilities and tasks improve?

Answer: _____

_____

_____

_____

Self-Care and Wellness:

Question: How would your self-care practices and overall wellness routine be affected?

Answer: _____

_____

_____

_____

Spiritual Connection:

Question: How would your spiritual life and sense of inner peace be enhanced?

Answer: _____
_____
_____
_____

Deep Reflection:

✧ Envisioning the Healed You:
- Take a moment to write down a vivid description of the most healed version of yourself. What does this version of you look like, what does this version of you feel like, and how does this version of you act like?

_____
_____
_____
_____
_____
_____
_____
_____
_____
_____
_____
_____
_____

FROM CURSED TO CURED

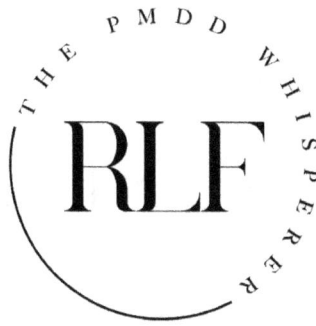

treating the root cause of PMDD one cycle at a time

Join the conversation about PMDD • Subconscious Mind • Neuroscience • RTT • Root Cause • Mind/Body/Spirit

@RACHELLYNNFOX

RACHEL LYNN FOX- THE PMDD WHISPERER: TREAT & CURE NATURALLY

@THEPMDDWHISPERER

I invite you to join my private Facebook Group: Treat & Cure PMDD Naturally.

APPENDIX

CHAPTER 2: THE MENSTRUAL CYCLE: A SHARED GLOBAL EXPERIENCE

1. "At any given moment, around 300 million women worldwide are sharing a common experience—menstruation, or as it's more casually known, having a period." - UNICEF Menstrual Health and Hygiene
2. "The average woman will ovulate about 300 to 400 times in her lifetime." - Cleveland Clinic: Menstrual Cycle Basics

The U.S. Perspective

3. "In the United States, there are roughly 166 million women, and about 64 million of them are in the menstruating age range of 12-49." - US Census Bureau
4. "The average American woman will have about 450 periods in her lifetime, which adds up to roughly 6.25 years of menstruating." - American College of Obstetricians and Gynecologists (ACOG)
5. "Over her lifetime, a woman might use between 11,000 to 16,000 tampons or pads." - National Institute of Environmental Health Sciences (NIEHS)
6. "Each month, your body conducts an intricate hormonal symphony, with estrogen, progesterone, FSH, and LH all taking turns in the spotlight." - Hormone Health Network
7. "The average menstrual cycle is about 28 days, but cycles ranging from 21 to 35 days are perfectly normal." - Mayo Clinic
8. "The U.S. menstrual products market is worth over $3 billion annually." - Market Research Reports
9. "The average age for a girl to get her first period in the U.S. is around 12." - Centers for Disease Control and Prevention (CDC)

10. "Approximately 75% of women experience some form of premenstrual syndrome (PMS)." - Office on Women's Health
11. "Menstrual cups and reusable pads are becoming increasingly popular in the U.S." - Journal of Women's Health
12. "Around 1 in 5 girls in the U.S. have missed school due to a lack of access to menstrual products." - Period.org
13. "A few progressive companies in the U.S. are starting to offer menstrual leave policies." - Forbes

Getting to Know the Phases of the Menstrual Cycle

14. "The menstrual cycle's connection to the seasons and lunar cycles offers profound insights into the natural rhythms that govern our lives." - International Journal of Environmental Research and Public Health
15. "Women gathered in 'moon lodges' or 'red tents' to honor their cycles." - The Red Tent Movement

Phases of the Menstrual Cycle: Detailed Information

16. Menstruation Phase: "Estrogen and Progesterone are at their lowest levels." - Cleveland Clinic: Menstrual Cycle Basics
17. Follicular Phase: "Estrogen levels begin to rise, promoting the thickening of the endometrial lining." - American College of Obstetricians and Gynecologists (ACOG)
18. Ovulation Phase: "LH surges to trigger the release of the mature egg from the ovary." - Mayo Clinic
19. Luteal Phase: "Progesterone levels rise, preparing the endometrial lining for potential implantation of a fertilized egg." - National Institute of Health (NIH)

Hormones Involved in the Menstrual Cycle

20. "The pituitary gland, often termed the 'master gland,' is a small, pea-sized organ located at the base of the brain." - Hormone Health Network
21. "The hypothalamus releases GnRH, which signals the pituitary gland to release FSH and LH." - Endocrine Society

22. "Estrogen, primarily produced during the follicular phase, helps to thicken the uterine lining (endometrium)." - National Institute of Environmental Health Sciences (NIEHS)
23. "Progesterone, produced by the corpus luteum after ovulation, further prepares the endometrium for potential implantation of a fertilized egg." - American Society for Reproductive Medicine (ASRM)

Supporting Hormonal Health

24. "Balanced Diet: Eating a variety of fruits, vegetables, whole grains, and lean proteins supports overall health." - Harvard T.H. Chan School of Public Health
25. "Regular Exercise: Engaging in moderate physical activity helps regulate hormones and reduce stress." - American Heart Association
26. "Quality Sleep: Aim for 7-9 hours of quality sleep per night." - National Sleep Foundation

The Endocrine System and Its Role

27. "The endocrine system is a complex network of glands that produce, store, and release hormones." - Mayo Clinic
28. "The hypothalamus plays a crucial role in maintaining homeostasis by linking the nervous system to the endocrine system." - Endocrine Society

Early Detection Through Awareness

29. "Understanding the phases and hormones of the menstrual cycle empowers women to recognize patterns in their symptoms." - Journal of Women's Health

Breaking the Silence: A Personal Reflection

30. "For centuries, women's health, especially regarding menstrual cycles, has been cloaked in silence and stigma." - National Women's Health Network

Global Impact of Menstrual Cycle Education

31. "In many developed countries, menstrual cycle education is integrated into school curriculums." - UNESCO

32. "In many developing countries, menstrual cycle education is often insufficient or entirely absent." - UNICEF
33. "Cultural beliefs and practices significantly shape how menstruation is perceived and managed." - World Health Organization (WHO)

CHAPTER 3: UNDERSTANDING PMDD: WHAT IS PMDD?

1. American Psychiatric Association. (2013). *Diagnostic and Statistical Manual of Mental Disorders (DSM-5)*. American Psychiatric Publishing.
2. International Association for Premenstrual Disorders (IAPMD). PMDD Facts and Statistics. Retrieved from IAPMD
3. Yonkers, K. A., O'Brien, P. M., & Eriksson, E. (2008). Premenstrual syndrome. *The Lancet, 371*(9619), 1200-1210.
4. The statistic that "1 in 12 women" suffer from Premenstrual Dysphoric Disorder (PMDD) is mentioned in several health sources. Verywell Health IAPMD

PMDD Symptoms and Personal Impact

5. Biggs, W. S., & Demuth, R. H. (2011). Premenstrual syndrome and premenstrual dysphoric disorder. *American Family Physician, 84*(8), 918-924.
6. Freeman, E. W., Halbreich, U., Grubb, G. S., Rapkin, A., & Yonkers, K. A. (2004). Reproductive hormones and PMS: Mood and cognitive function. *Obstetrics & Gynecology Clinics of North America, 31*(3), 219-239.
7. Pearlstein, T., & Steiner, M. (2008). Premenstrual dysphoric disorder: Burden of illness and treatment update. *Journal of Psychiatry & Neuroscience, 33*(4), 291-301.

PMDD Causes: Traditional and Holistic Perspectives

8. Schmidt, P. J., & Rubinow, D. R. (1997). Sex hormones and mood in the perimenopause. *Annals of the New York Academy of Sciences, 828*(1), 70-82.
9. Yonkers, K. A., Pearlstein, T. B., Foegh, M., Brown, C., Sampson-Landers, C., & Rapkin, A. (2005). Efficacy of a new low-dose

oral contraceptive with drospirenone in premenstrual dysphoric disorder. *Obstetrics & Gynecology, 106*(3), 492-501.

10. Girdler, S. S., & Klatzkin, R. R. (2007). Biological responses to stress in premenstrual dysphoric disorder: Influence of history of depression and anxiety, response to stressors, and functional status. *Psychoneuroendocrinology, 32*(7), 667-679.

11. International Association for Premenstrual Disorders (IAPMD). (2018). PMDD and Suicide. Retrieved from IAPMD

Traditional and Holistic Treatments for PMDD

12. Pearlstein, T. (2016). Treatment of premenstrual dysphoric disorder: Therapeutic challenges. *Expert Review of Clinical Pharmacology, 9*(4), 493-502.

13. Steiner, M., Streiner, D. L., & Soares, C. N. (2008). Management of premenstrual symptoms and premenstrual dysphoric disorder. *Psychopharmacology Bulletin, 41*(1), 5-30.

14. Bäckström, T., Haage, D., Löfgren, M., Johansson, I. M., Strömberg, J., Nyberg, S., & Andréen, L. (2014). Neurosteroids—Effects on mood, cognition and memory. *Psychoneuroendocrinology, 42*(1), 36-46.

15. Roca, C. A., Schmidt, P. J., & Rubinow, D. R. (1999). A follow-up study of premenstrual syndrome in adolescence. *Journal of Clinical Psychiatry, 60*(3), 172-177.

Impact of PMDD on Daily Life and Relationships

16. Dennerstein, L., Lehert, P., & Bäckström, T. (2010). Premenstrual symptoms—severity, duration and typology: An international cross-sectional study. *Menopause International, 16*(3), 120-126.

17. Reid, R. L., & Yen, S. S. (1981). Premenstrual syndrome. *American Journal of Obstetrics and Gynecology, 139*(1), 85-104.

18. The American College of Obstetricians and Gynecologists (ACOG). (2015). Premenstrual Syndrome (PMS). Retrieved from ACOG

Recognition of PMDD in DSM-5 and Suicidal Risks

19. American Psychiatric Association. (2013). Diagnostic and Statistical Manual of Mental Disorders (DSM-5). American Psychiatric Publishing.

20. Epperson, C. N., Steiner, M., & Hartlage, S. A. (2012). Premenstrual dysphoric disorder: Evidence for a new category for DSM-5. *American Journal of Psychiatry, 169*(5), 465-475.
21. International Association for Premenstrual Disorders (IAPMD). (2018). PMDD and Suicide. Retrieved from IAPMD

Diagnosis Journey and Symptom Tracking

22. Halbreich, U. (2003). The diagnosis of premenstrual syndromes and premenstrual dysphoric disorder—clinical procedures and research perspectives. *Gynecological Endocrinology, 17*(3), 25-36.
23. Rapkin, A. J., & Winer, S. A. (2009). Premenstrual syndrome and premenstrual dysphoric disorder: Quality of life and burden of illness. *Expert Review of Pharmacoeconomics & Outcomes Research, 9*(2), 157-170.
24. International Association for Premenstrual Disorders (IAPMD). (2021). Diagnostic Criteria for PMDD. Retrieved from IAPMD
25. International Association for Premenstrual Disorders (IAPMD). (2019). Symptom Tracking for PMDD. Retrieved from IAPMD

CHAPTER 4: LIVING WITH PREMENSTRUAL DYSPHORIC DISORDER (PMDD)

1. Halbreich, U., Borenstein, J., Pearlstein, T., & Kahn, L. S. (2003). The prevalence, impairment, impact, and burden of premenstrual dysphoric disorder (PMS/PMDD). *Psychoneuroendocrinology, 28*(3), 1-23.
2. American Psychiatric Association. (2013). *Diagnostic and Statistical Manual of Mental Disorders (DSM-5)*. American Psychiatric Publishing.
3. Yonkers, K. A., O'Brien, P. M., & Eriksson, E. (2008). Premenstrual syndrome. *The Lancet, 371*(9619), 1200-1210.

Victimhood Consciousness

4. Schwartz, G. E., & Rogers, J. (2001). Self-blame and distress among women with premenstrual dysphoric disorder. *Journal of Clinical Psychology, 57*(12), 1445-1457.
5. Alloy, L. B., Abramson, L. Y., Hogan, M. E., Whitehouse, W. G., Rose, D. T., Robinson, M. S., & Kim, R. S. (2000). The Temple-Wisconsin Cognitive Vulnerability to Depression (CVD) Project: Lifetime histo-

ry of Axis I psychopathology in individuals at high and low cognitive risk for depression. *Journal of Abnormal Psychology, 109*(3), 403-418.

Signs of Victim Consciousness

6. Seligman, M. E. P. (1975). *Helplessness: On Depression, Development, and Death.* W.H. Freeman.
7. Koss, M. P., & Figueredo, A. J. (2004). Change in cognitive mediators of rape's impact on psychosocial health across 2 years of recovery. *Journal of Consulting and Clinical Psychology, 72*(6), 1063-1072.
8. Janoff-Bulman, R. (1992). *Shattered Assumptions: Towards a New Psychology of Trauma.* Free Press.

Negative Self-Talk and Cognitive Behavioral Therapy

9. Beck, A. T. (1976). *Cognitive Therapy and the Emotional Disorders.* International Universities Press.
10. Ellis, A. (2001). *Feeling Better, Getting Better, Staying Better: Profound Self-Help Therapy for Your Emotions.* Impact Publishers.

Proactive Strategies for Empowerment

11. Neff, K. D. (2003). The development and validation of a scale to measure self-compassion. *Self and Identity, 2*(3), 223-250.
12. Kabat-Zinn, J. (1990). *Full Catastrophe Living: Using the Wisdom of Your Body and Mind to Face Stress, Pain, and Illness.* Delacorte.
13. Seligman, M. E. P. (2011). *Flourish: A Visionary New Understanding of Happiness and Well-being.* Free Press.
14. Shapiro, S. L., Carlson, L. E., Astin, J. A., & Freedman, B. (2006). Mechanisms of mindfulness. *Journal of Clinical Psychology, 62*(3), 373-386.
15. Lyubomirsky, S., King, L., & Diener, E. (2005). The benefits of frequent positive affect: Does happiness lead to success? *Psychological Bulletin, 131*(6), 803-855.

Transitioning from Victimhood to Empowerment

16. Frankl, V. E. (1984). *Man's Search for Meaning.* Beacon Press.
17. Csikszentmihalyi, M. (1990). *Flow: The Psychology of Optimal Experience.* Harper & Row.

18. Goleman, D. (1995). *Emotional Intelligence: Why It Can Matter More Than IQ*. Bantam Books.

CHAPTER 5: NAVIGATING THE TWO ROADS: THE NEXT CHAPTER IN YOUR PMDD JOURNEY

1. Frost, R. (1916). *The Road Not Taken*. In *Mountain Interval*. Henry Holt and Company.
2. Halbreich, U., Borenstein, J., Pearlstein, T., & Kahn, L. S. (2003). The prevalence, impairment, impact, and burden of premenstrual dysphoric disorder (PMS/PMDD). *Psychoneuroendocrinology, 28*(3), 1-23.
3. American Psychiatric Association. (2013). *Diagnostic and Statistical Manual of Mental Disorders (DSM-5)*. American Psychiatric Publishing.

Embracing the Journey of Ownership

4. Seligman, M. E. P. (1975). *Helplessness: On Depression, Development, and Death*. W.H. Freeman.
5. Janoff-Bulman, R. (1992). *Shattered Assumptions: Towards a New Psychology of Trauma*. Free Press.

The Wisdom of the Luteal Phase

6. Yonkers, K. A., O'Brien, P. M., & Eriksson, E. (2008). Premenstrual syndrome. *The Lancet, 371*(9619), 1200-1210.
7. van der Kolk, B. (2014). *The Body Keeps the Score: Brain, Mind, and Body in the Healing of Trauma*. Viking.

Understanding Trauma and Its Impact

8. Maté, G. (2003). *When the Body Says No: Exploring the Stress-Disease Connection*. Wiley.
9. Levine, P. A. (1997). *Waking the Tiger: Healing Trauma*. North Atlantic Books.

Recognizing Patterns and Themes

10. Neff, K. D. (2003). The development and validation of a scale to measure self-compassion. *Self and Identity, 2*(3), 223-250.

11. Kabat-Zinn, J. (1990). *Full Catastrophe Living: Using the Wisdom of Your Body and Mind to Face Stress, Pain, and Illness.* Delacorte.

Understanding Trauma Responses

12. Schore, A. N. (2003). *Affect Dysregulation and Disorders of the Self.* W.W. Norton & Company.
13. van der Kolk, B. (2014). *The Body Keeps the Score: Brain, Mind, and Body in the Healing of Trauma.* Viking.

Nervous System Dysregulation

14. Sapolsky, R. M. (2004). *Why Zebras Don't Get Ulcers.* Holt Paperbacks.
15. Porges, S. W. (2011). *The Polyvagal Theory: Neurophysiological Foundations of Emotions, Attachment, Communication, and Self-regulation.* W.W. Norton & Company.

Mindfulness and Meditation

16. Kabat-Zinn, J. (1994). *Wherever You Go, There You Are: Mindfulness Meditation in Everyday Life.* Hyperion.
17. Davidson, R. J., & McEwen, B. S. (2012). Social influences on neuroplasticity: Stress and interventions to promote well-being. *Nature Neuroscience, 15*(5), 689-695.

Somatic Practices for Healing

18. Levine, P. A. (1997). *Waking the Tiger: Healing Trauma.* North Atlantic Books.
19. van der Kolk, B. (2014). *The Body Keeps the Score: Brain, Mind, and Body in the Healing of Trauma.* Viking.

Nutrition and Lifestyle for Nervous System Health

20. Weil, A. (2004). *Healthy Aging: A Lifelong Guide to Your Well-Being.* Knopf.
21. Ramsay, J. R. (2009). *The Adrenal Reset Diet: Strategically Cycle Carbs and Proteins to Lose Weight, Balance Hormones, and Move from Stressed to Thriving.* Harmony.

CHAPTER 6: THE SENSITIVITY WITHIN

1. Aron, E. N. (1996). *The Highly Sensitive Person: How to Thrive When the World Overwhelms You.* Broadway Books.
2. Zeff, A. (2004). *The Highly Sensitive Person's Survival Guide: Essential Skills for Living Well in an Overstimulating World.* New Harbinger Publications.
3. Maté, G. (2003). *When the Body Says No: Exploring the Stress-Disease Connection.* Wiley.
4. Aron, E. N., & Aron, A. (1997). Sensory-processing sensitivity and its relation to introversion and emotionality. *Journal of Personality and Social Psychology, 73*(2), 345-368.
5. Elaine Aron, "The Highly Sensitive Person: Stress and Health," https://hsperson.com/ (accessed August 5, 2024).

Sensitivity in Childhood and Personality Types

6. Jung, C. G. (1971). *Psychological Types.* Princeton University Press.
7. Myers, I. B., & Myers, P. B. (1995). *Gifts Differing: Understanding Personality Type.* Davies-Black Publishing.
8. Nardi, D. (2010). *Neuroscience of Personality: Brain Savvy Insights for All Types of People.* Radiance House.

Highly Sensitive Persons (HSPs)

9. Aron, E. N. (2010). *Psychotherapy and the Highly Sensitive Person: Improving Outcomes for That Minority of People Who Are the Majority of Clients.* Routledge.
10. Kagan, J., & Snidman, N. (2004). *The Long Shadow of Temperament.* Harvard University Press.

Hormonal Influences on Sensitivity

11. Schore, A. N. (2012). *The Science of the Art of Psychotherapy.* W.W. Norton & Company.
12. Brizendine, L. (2006). *The Female Brain.* Broadway Books.
13. Schmidt, P. J., & Rubinow, D. R. (1991). Neuroregulation of mood: Implications for understanding the pathogenesis of PMDD. *Journal of Clinical Endocrinology and Metabolism, 73*(1), 149-158.

Sensitivity and Mental Health

14. van der Kolk, B. (2014). *The Body Keeps the Score: Brain, Mind, and Body in the Healing of Trauma.* Viking.

15. Porges, S. W. (2011). *The Polyvagal Theory: Neurophysiological Foundations of Emotions, Attachment, Communication, and Self-regulation.* W.W. Norton & Company.

16. Gilbert, P. (2010). *The Compassionate Mind: A New Approach to Life's Challenges.* New Harbinger Publications.

Mind-Body Connection

17. Kabat-Zinn, J. (1990). *Full Catastrophe Living: Using the Wisdom of Your Body and Mind to Face Stress, Pain, and Illness.* Delacorte.

18. Siegel, D. J. (2012). *The Developing Mind: How Relationships and the Brain Interact to Shape Who We Are.* Guilford Press.

Honoring Sensitivity and Personal Growth

19. Neff, K. D. (2011). *Self-Compassion: The Proven Power of Being Kind to Yourself.* William Morrow.

20. Brown, B. (2012). *Daring Greatly: How the Courage to Be Vulnerable Transforms the Way We Live, Love, Parent, and Lead.* Gotham Books.

Sensitivity and Creativity

21. Kaufman, S. B., & Gregoire, C. (2015). *Wired to Create: Unraveling the Mysteries of the Creative Mind.* Perigee Books.

22. Csikszentmihalyi, M. (1996). *Creativity: Flow and the Psychology of Discovery and Invention.* HarperCollins.

Understanding and Managing PMDD

23. Hantsoo, L., & Epperson, C. N. (2015). Premenstrual Dysphoric Disorder: Epidemiology and Treatment. *Current Psychiatry Reports, 17*(11), 87.

24. Yonkers, K. A., O'Brien, P. M., & Eriksson, E. (2008). Premenstrual syndrome. *The Lancet, 371*(9619), 1200-1210.

25. Rapkin, A. J., & Winer, S. A. (2009). Premenstrual Dysphoric Disorder: Pathophysiology and Treatment Approaches. *Obstetrics and Gynecology Clinics of North America, 36*(4), 907-924.

CHAPTER 7: UNDERSTANDING SYMPTOMS AS MESSENGERS

Listening to the Body's Messages

1. Mate, G. (2003). *When the Body Says No: Exploring the Stress-Disease Connection.* Wiley.
2. Pert, C. B. (1997). *Molecules of Emotion: The Science Behind Mind-Body Medicine.* Scribner.

Decoding the Language of Symptoms 3. Scaer, R. C. (2005). *The Trauma Spectrum: Hidden Wounds and Human Resiliency.* W.W. Norton & Company. 4. Levine, P. A. (2010). *In an Unspoken Voice: How the Body Releases Trauma and Restores Goodness.* North Atlantic Books.

The Nature of Triggers 5. van der Kolk, B. A. (2014). *The Body Keeps the Score: Brain, Mind, and Body in the Healing of Trauma.* Viking. 6. Sapolsky, R. M. (2004). *Why Zebras Don't Get Ulcers: The Acclaimed Guide to Stress, Stress-Related Diseases, and Coping.* Holt Paperbacks.

Connecting Triggers to PMDD Symptoms 7. Yonkers, K. A., & O'Brien, P. M. S. (2008). Premenstrual syndrome. *The Lancet, 371*(9619), 1200-1210. 8. Schmidt, P. J., & Rubinow, D. R. (1991). Neuroregulation of mood: Implications for understanding the pathogenesis of PMDD. *Journal of Clinical Endocrinology and Metabolism, 73*(1), 149-158.

Example 1: Dinner Disagreement and Example 2: Career Critique 9. Linehan, M. M. (1993). *Cognitive-Behavioral Treatment of Borderline Personality Disorder.* The Guilford Press. 10. Bowlby, J. (1988). *A Secure Base: Parent-Child Attachment and Healthy Human Development.* Basic Books.

What Is Our Mind and Body Revealing? 11. Kabat-Zinn, J. (1990). *Full Catastrophe Living: Using the Wisdom of Your Body and Mind to Face Stress, Pain, and Illness.* Delacorte. 12. Neff, K. D. (2011). *Self-Compassion: The Proven Power of Being Kind to Yourself.* William Morrow.

The Luteal Phase as a Revealer of the Subconscious 13. Schore, A. N. (2012). *The Science of the Art of Psychotherapy.* W.W. Norton & Company. 14. Luyten, P., Mayes, L. C., Fonagy, P., & Target, M. (2007). The emotional foundation of human personality. *Neuroscience and Biobehavioral Reviews, 31*(7), 1007-1017.

The Formation and Power of the Subconscious Mind 15. Montessori, M. (1967). *The Absorbent Mind.* Holt, Rinehart and Winston. 16. Siegel, D. J. (2012). *The Developing Mind: How Relationships and the Brain Interact to Shape Who We Are.* Guilford Press.

The Subconscious Mind's Protective Role 17. Perry, B. D., & Szalavitz, M. (2017). *The Boy Who Was Raised as a Dog: And Other Stories from a Child Psychiatrist's Notebook--What Traumatized Children Can Teach Us About Loss, Love, and Healing.* Basic Books. 18. Rothschild, B. (2000). *The Body Remembers: The Psychophysiology of Trauma and Trauma Treatment.* W.W. Norton & Company.

Understanding the Four Trauma Responses 19. Herman, J. L. (1992). *Trauma and Recovery: The Aftermath of Violence--From Domestic Abuse to Political Terror.* Basic Books. 20. Ogden, P., Minton, K., & Pain, C. (2006). *Trauma and the Body: A Sensorimotor Approach to Psychotherapy.* W.W. Norton & Company.

Integration and Moving Forward: Embracing Healing and Growth 21. Siegel, D. J., & Solomon, M. F. (2003). *Healing Trauma: Attachment, Mind, Body and Brain.* W.W. Norton & Company. 22. Porges, S. W. (2011). *The Polyvagal Theory: Neurophysiological Foundations of Emotions, Attachment, Communication, and Self-Regulation.* W.W. Norton & Company.

CHAPTER 8: THE DEEP DIVE

Awakening to the Root Cause of PMDD

1. Yonkers, K. A., & O'Brien, P. M. S. (2008). Premenstrual syndrome. *The Lancet, 371*(9619), 1200-1210.

2. Schmidt, P. J., & Rubinow, D. R. (1991). Neuroregulation of mood: Implications for understanding the pathogenesis of PMDD. *Journal of Clinical Endocrinology and Metabolism, 73*(1), 149-158.

Understanding the Subconscious and Emotional Pain 3. Pert, C. B. (1997). *Molecules of Emotion: The Science Behind Mind-Body Medicine.* Scribner. 4. Mate, G. (2003). *When the Body Says No: Exploring the Stress-Disease Connection.* Wiley.

The Subconscious Mind and Childhood Experiences 5. Montessori, M. (1967). *The Absorbent Mind*. Holt, Rinehart and Winston. 6. Siegel, D. J. (2012). *The Developing Mind: How Relationships and the Brain Interact to Shape Who We Are*. Guilford Press. 7. Perry, B. D., & Szalavitz, M. (2017). *The Boy Who Was Raised as a Dog: And Other Stories from a Child Psychiatrist's Notebook--What Traumatized Children Can Teach Us About Loss, Love, and Healing*. Basic Books.

Neuroplasticity and Changing Beliefs 8. Doidge, N. (2007). *The Brain That Changes Itself: Stories of Personal Triumph from the Frontiers of Brain Science*. Penguin Books. 9. Schwartz, J. M., & Begley, S. (2003). *The Mind and the Brain: Neuroplasticity and the Power of Mental Force*. Harper Perennial.

The Gut-Brain Connection 10. Mayer, E. A. (2016). *The Mind-Gut Connection: How the Hidden Conversation Within Our Bodies Impacts Our Mood, Our Choices, and Our Overall Health*. Harper Wave. 11. Cryan, J. F., & Dinan, T. G. (2012). Mind-altering microorganisms: The impact of the gut microbiota on brain and behavior. *Nature Reviews Neuroscience, 13*(10), 701-712.

Rapid Transformational Therapy (RTT) 12. Peer, M. (2018). *I Am Enough: Mark Your Mirror And Change Your Life*. Piatkus. 13. Yapko, M. D. (2011). *Trancework: An Introduction to the Practice of Clinical Hypnosis*. Routledge. 14. Rossi, E. L. (2002). *The Psychobiology of Gene Expression: Neuroscience and Neurogenesis in Hypnosis and the Healing Arts*. W.W. Norton & Company.

Hypnotherapy and Cognitive Behavioral Therapy (CBT) 15. Butler, G., & McManus, F. (2007). Psychology: A very short introduction. *Oxford University Press*. 16. Burns, D. D. (1980). *Feeling Good: The New Mood Therapy*. William Morrow & Company.

Inner Child Healing and Subconscious Beliefs 17. Schore, A. N. (2012). *The Science of the Art of Psychotherapy*. W.W. Norton & Company. 18. Herman, J. L. (1992). *Trauma and Recovery: The Aftermath of Violence--From Domestic Abuse to Political Terror*. Basic Books.

Scientific Validation and Personal Testimonials 19. van der Kolk, B. A. (2014). *The Body Keeps the Score: Brain, Mind, and Body in the Healing of Trauma*. Viking. 20. Neff, K. D. (2011). *Self-Compassion: The Proven Power of Being Kind to Yourself*. William Morrow.

CHAPTER 9: YOUR HIGHER SELF IS CALLING

Reclaiming Your True Self: Beyond the Shadows of PMDD

The Call to Reclaim Your Identity

1. Greco, T., & Herbst, K. L. (2017). PMDD: Understanding and Treating Premenstrual Dysphoric Disorder. *Women's Health*, 13(3), 1-12.
2. Steiner, M., & Pearlstein, T. (2000). Premenstrual Dysphoric Disorder: Burden of Illness and Treatment Update. *Journal of Psychiatry & Neuroscience*, 25(5), 459-468.

Awakening Your Highest Self 3. Beck, J. S. (2011). *Cognitive Behavior Therapy: Basics and Beyond*. Guilford Press. 4. Brown, B. (2010). *The Gifts of Imperfection: Let Go of Who You Think You're Supposed to Be and Embrace Who You Are*. Hazelden Publishing.

The Journey Beyond Pain 5. Levine, P. A. (1997). *Waking the Tiger: Healing Trauma*. North Atlantic Books. 6. Maté, G. (2010). *In the Realm of Hungry Ghosts: Close Encounters with Addiction*. Vintage Canada.

Embracing Your New Reality 7. Kabat-Zinn, J. (1990). *Full Catastrophe Living: Using the Wisdom of Your Body and Mind to Face Stress, Pain, and Illness*. Delacorte Press. 8. Bowlby, J. (1988). *A Secure Base: Parent-Child Attachment and Healthy Human Development*. Basic Books.

Stepping into Your Light 9. Siegel, D. J., & Bryson, T. P. (2011). *The Whole-Brain Child: 12 Revolutionary Strategies to Nurture Your Child's Developing Mind*. Delacorte Press. 10. Neff, K. (2011). *Self-Compassion: The Proven Power of Being Kind to Yourself*. William Morrow.

Insights from Scriptures 11. The Holy Bible, New International Version. (1978). *Zondervan Publishing House*.

Spiritual Laws and Higher Self 12. Byrne, R. (2006). *The Secret*. Atria Books. 13. Hicks, E., & Hicks, J. (2006). *The Law of Attraction: The Basics of the Teachings of Abraham*. Hay House Inc. 14. Tolle, E. (2005). *A New Earth: Awakening to Your Life's Purpose*. Penguin Group.

Science of Light: Quantum Physics and Neuroscience 15. Dispenza, J. (2012). *Breaking the Habit of Being Yourself: How to Lose Your Mind and Create a New One*. Hay House Inc. 16. Capra, F. (1982). *The Turning Point: Science, Society, and the Rising Culture*. Bantam Books. 17. Kandel, E.

R. (2006). *In Search of Memory: The Emergence of a New Science of Mind.* W.W. Norton & Company.

The Road to Evolving and Ascension 18. Lipton, B. H. (2005). *The Biology of Belief: Unleashing the Power of Consciousness, Matter, & Miracles.* Hay House Inc. 19. Wilber, K. (2000). *A Brief History of Everything.* Shambhala Publications.

Ongoing Journey 20. Chopra, D. (2009). *Reinventing the Body, Resurrecting the Soul: How to Create a New You.* Harmony. 21. Myss, C. (2006). *Entering the Castle: An Inner Path to God and Your Soul.* Free Press.

Call to Remember Who You Are 22. Emmons, H. (2006). *The Chemistry of Calm: A Powerful, Drug-Free Plan to Quiet Your Fears and Overcome Your Anxiety.* Touchstone. 23. Williamson, M. (1992). *A Return to Love: Reflections on the Principles of "A Course in Miracles".* HarperOne.

ABOUT THE AUTHOR

Rachel Lynn Fox, known as The PMDD Whisperer, is a certified Rapid Transformational Therapy (RTT) practitioner, spiritual guide, and advocate for women's health. Her healing journey began when she discovered she had premenstrual dysphoric disorder (PMDD) after suffering for 25 years with undiagnosed symptoms. After trying various traditional approaches, she found a root-cause solution through the transformative power of RTT, which allowed her to completely alleviate her PMDD symptoms and naturally cure her PMDD. This breakthrough inspired her to dedicate her life to helping others heal.

A New York City resident for over a decade, Rachel is a devoted wife, mother of two, stepmother of two, puppy mama, and spiritual seeker. Through her Living in Luteal programs and her Instagram account @rachellynnfox, she offers holistic and spiritual guidance for women to reconnect with their true selves and reclaim their lives from PMDD. Her work fosters hope, faith, and personal transformation, encouraging women to take charge of their healing journeys.

In her free time, Rachel cherishes moments with her family and friends and enjoys soaking up the vibrant energy of New York City. She also finds peace in Naples, Florida, where she enjoys the beach, swimming, and reconnecting with nature.

www.ingramcontent.com/pod-product-compliance
Lightning Source LLC
Chambersburg PA
CBHW051548020426
42333CB00016B/2153